IN BED ALONE

A Caregiver's Odyssey

by

LEN KREISLER, MD

Husband, father, physician

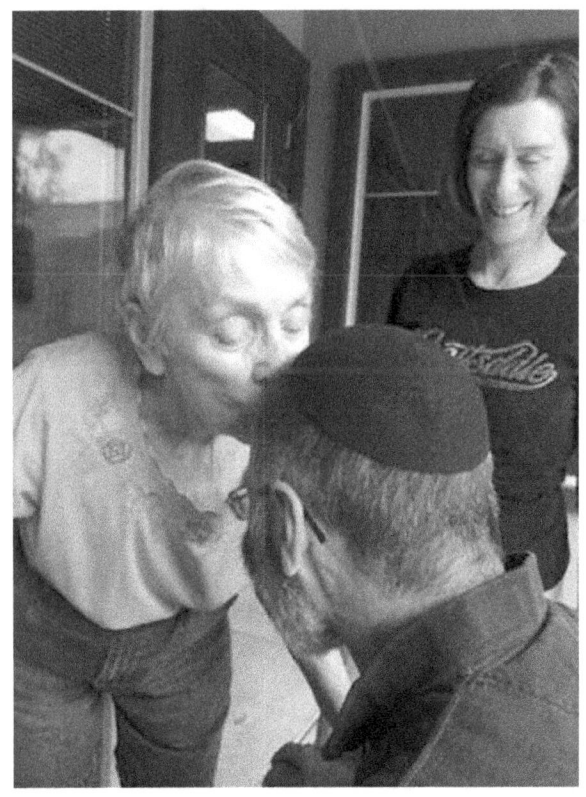

Some serenity, some sadness, lots of acceptance

Also by Len Kreisler, MD

Available from the author only:
Death by Any Means
(Terrorism, bacteria, political, America and world, novel)

Roll the Dice, Pick a Doc and Hope for the Best
(Medical nonfiction: health care in the United States)

The Codes of Babylon
(Medical novel: Las Vegas politics)

Shortfall
(Novel: politics, energy, and espionage)

The Obligated Volunteer
(Nonfiction: a medical/political/military memoir)

In Bed Alone

ISBN: 1533574537
ISBN 13: 9781533574534

DEDICATION

Remember the phrase "the grass appears greener in other people's yards"? While that may be a truthful perspective, reality tells us we all have challenges, from the moment of conception to our final breaths on earth. Philosophers give us their take on the facets of life, scientists strive to explain the "why's" and "how's" in factual terms, and spiritual leaders…well, a lot of comfort and a lot of tragedy emerges in humanity's struggle to give meaning for our existence here.

Some answers have evolved for me from all of the above. My parents fled Europe to a country founded on the principles of freedom and hope: work hard, play by the rules, and you will have a chance to learn, contribute, and enjoy the fruits of your labors. We have enjoyed the American Dream. I dedicate this book to all the families who have similarly experienced the dream of "milk and honey" in a land that is continuously struggling to make itself better.

The title page photo is more personal: my wife of over half a century and two of our three children caught in a visual moment impossible to describe by words alone. My wife, Joan, kissing our eldest son, Kevin, on the forehead as our daughter, Kay, beams with joy. Why is this situation so remarkable? Dr. Kevin Goeta Kreisler is a psychiatrist in nearby Tucson, Arizona. Kay Segal is an accomplished businesswoman in the convenience store industry living in Scottsdale, Arizona. Their mother has had a history of progressive cognitive impairment for over ten years. A year before this photo was taken, Joan fell and fractured her right wrist and right hip. After her acute rehabilitation, it was obvious that I could not continue with home care where we lived in Las Vegas. She was in a group home for six months and then moved to a memory care facility close to our daughter in Scottsdale. Kevin has been part of her medical team, and this photo was taken while he was reviewing her medications and medical progress and simply visiting to comfort his mother. Our youngest son, Kenneth, an anesthesiologist at the University of Kansas Hospital (also known as KU-Med) in Kansas City, has also been involved with his mother's care and comfort. As you can imagine, Joan has indeed lost a good share of her ability to comprehend and express thoughts and emotions. As seen in the photo, however, the family bonds persist despite the challenges involved. We are indeed fortunate to be able to provide peace of mind and a supportive environment for Joan: an environment that also includes periodic visits and bonding with all eight of our grandchildren.

I am deeply indebted to our children for their support and understanding. Joan and I did put a lot of time and effort into doing the best we could with family values and day-to-day challenges. We recognize the added element of luck. We're proud of their personal accomplishments and contributions to society. I'm particularly indebted to Kay Segal's editing and prodding to "get it done" and for Howard Segal's time and expertise with computer technology. Without the assistance of both of them, this book might never have been written.

Some serenity, some sadness, lots of acceptance.

Contents

PREFACE WHEN YOUR WORLD GOES QUIET, THE BRAIN
STRUGGLES TO SURVIVE   VII

CHAPT. I UNDERSTANDING WORDS   1
CHAPT. II A FEW FACES OF DEMENTIA   13
CHAPT. III TRANSPARENCY AND ACCOUNTABILITY   29
CHAPT. IV PERCEPTIONS AND BEHAVIOR—EACH CASE
UNTO ITSELF   43
CHAPT. V IS IT JUST SOMETHING AGE APPROPRIATE?   55
CHAPT. VI EMOTIONS, FACTS, AND DENIALS   67
CHAPT. VII DOING GOOD TAKES GRIT   77
CHAPT. VIII THE NAKED TRUTH   87
CHAPT. IX ACUTE CARE, PALLIATIVE CARE, HOSPICE CARE   95
CHAPT. X ONE FROM THE HEART   97

EPILOGUE   109
REFERENCES AND FURTHER READING   111
ABOUT THE AUTHOR   123

WHEN YOUR WORLD GOES QUIET, THE BRAIN STRUGGLES TO SURVIVE

Finding out you or a loved one has a medical issue is like David facing Goliath with nothing but his loincloth. Being a physician gave me some advantages, but the journey still proved to be a daily learning experience. Sharing my challenges and attempts to cope with limited options will, I hope, help others get the answers they need for dealing with current demands and anticipating future choices.

Joan and I were married in 1957, the year I graduated from the University of Vermont College Of Medicine. Joan had graduated in 1956 with a BA degree; she went on to get a master's in teaching at Columbia University in New York City while I completed my senior year of medical school. We were married at her aunt's house in Connecticut right after completion of medical school but before the actual graduation ceremony in Vermont. After our marriage, she taught biology at the very upscale Scarsdale High School in Westchester County, New York. We lived in the nearby county hospital officially called Grasslands Hospital, Valhalla, New York. The resident and intern staff had their own quarters, dining room and lounge in the main hospital building. Joan and I had one room and a shared bath with another couple. Upon completion of my internship at the County Hospital, I took and passed Part III of the National Board Exams at Yale University. In those days most MD (allopathic) physicians took the three part National Board exams: Part I after the first two years of medical school, Part II upon graduation from school, Part III upon completion of a post graduate training program. To be eligible for licensing as a family physician in those states accepting the National Boards, I took one year of a rotating medical internship which is not available any more. To be licensed for family practice now requires a three year approved residency program. Surgery, and other specialties had several-year residency programs, as they do to this day.

I was then licensed to practice medicine and surgery in the state of New York. Since physicians were eligible for the draft up to age thirty-six, and I was only twenty-eight, I, like many others, opted to volunteer for my two-year service obligation, thus avoiding being called out of an established medical practice at a later time for a national emergency.

Everything went well with my military indoctrination at Fort Sam Houston in San Antonio, Texas. My subsequent assignment to Fort Detrick, Maryland, for bacteriologic warfare research, and later (at my request) to Fort Ritchie, Maryland ("Site R"), as post surgeon, were both growth experiences. Site R is nicknamed the "Underground Pentagon," because the hollowed-out mountain is intended to serve as a command-and-control center in time of national crises. Indeed, that is where Vice President Dick Cheney was allegedly sent on 9/11. My military experience is revealed in detail in my book *The Obligated Volunteer*, available at CreateSpace.com. It was not the run-of-the-mill tour of duty, and I loved it. Had I been single, I most likely would have made a career of it. It was lucky for me that Fort Detrick was only an hour or so away from Walter Reed Army Hospital in Washington, DC, directly under the command of the army surgeon general. At Fort Detrick, Joan went into a full-blown manic episode; right out of the blue. I knew that her father and brother were diagnosed with the disease and that they had numerous electroshock treatments for recurrent manic episodes. There were no definitive medications. We called it manic-depressive disease in those days. It later became known as bipolar disease. I might have gotten a few-sentence mention of the disease in my training, but it wasn't a factor in our falling in love.

That day will never be forgotten. Joan's behavior became acutely irrational and exuberant, as if someone had given her a huge dose of adrenalin or amphetamines (or "uppers"). She couldn't sleep, concentrate, eat, or relate. I gave it a day or two before contacting Walter Reed and had her admitted. It was surreal; so overwhelming that I did not process the experience as happening to me and my relatively new wife. I was treating the situation as an abstract medical challenge, not something personal. This form of denial helped me move quickly and objectively to address the medical problem and not get hung up with emotional paralysis. Fortunately, a very well-qualified young psychiatrist at Walter Reed took charge of Joan's case. All expenses were covered, as was medical leave from my duties for as long as would be necessary.

Hope and denial may spring eternal, but reality is consistently present and sobering. There were only two options: electroshock therapy, with more rapid results, or chemotherapy (Thorazine), which could take a good four to six weeks. I had spent a month at the Brattleboro Retreat in Vermont, a psychiatric hospital, in my third year of medical school. It was an elective. I was very interested in psychology and human behavior from my first formal exposure to psychology as a freshman at Allegheny College, in Meadville, Pennsylvania.

Electroshock therapy at Brattleboro, as practiced in 1956, was more like watching prisoner interrogation. The patient was immobilized on a table and a bite-block placed in his or her mouth so as to avoid biting the tongue. A lot of electric current was given through electrodes placed on both sides of the head, which was combined with insulin shock (an injection of enough insulin to severely lower the patient's blood sugar). The combination caused violent seizures, loss of consciousness, and who knew what else. The patient was then placed in a bathtub filled with ice cubes. I can't remember what type of sedating medication was given prior to treatment—probably a barbiturate of some kind—but I'm sure the person was not in deep anesthesia. Patients were dazed or coma-like after treatment. They did not complain or seem to recall the ordeal. Our son, the psychiatrist in Tucson, tells me that today's ECT (electroconvulsive therapy) is very much gentler and very effective, especially with older people in a depressive state. It was shortly after admission to Walter Reed that I obtained Joan's full family history of her father's and brother's diagnosis of bipolar disease and the multiple shock treatments and whatever limited medications were available at the time. People didn't, and still don't, like to talk about mental diseases. Although the stigma is much less today than it once was (as it should be), shame, guilt, and misperceptions still hamper timely diagnosis, treatment, and discussions. I will get into definitions, case examples, and discussions of bipolar disease, dementias, movement disorders, and other neurologic challenges in the first chapter of this book.

I was very familiar with the use of Thorazine in my medical training and opted to have Joan treated with whatever amount of medication was necessary. I was not allowed to see or communicate with her until her treating physician thought she had adequately responded and was into her recovery phase, when she would experience a slow downward tapering of the dosage: usually three to four weeks. I understood the process very well, since it had been part of my training at the Brattleboro Retreat Psychiatric Hospital in Vermont. I also vividly recalled images of patients shuffling around like dazed zombies, with no sense of time, place, or person; the patient and physician would be in limbo as both waited for "chemical imbalances to normalize," as they would say. At the time it sounded like doctors like me really knew what we were talking about, but actually we knew very little and were good at sounding like we did. We knew the treatment worked to bring the patient out of manic behavior, but we had very little understanding of how or why. I sometimes get the same feeling as we struggle to understand current mental disease states.

Knowing too much can be agonizing when you are forced to choose a plan of action. I knew what the package insert said about unintended adverse reactions. I had not seen any problems firsthand, since in the early 1950s this was a relatively new choice of treatment for bipolar disease. I preferred to believe that I, as a doctor, could manage anything. Call it denial or selective arrogance, but I had participated in some very gratifying treatments during my training to be a physician and I somehow conveniently ignored the humbling failures I had witnessed. We had no Internet search engines at the time, of course, but we did have package inserts. Here's an example of the caveats, with excerpts paraphrased from Wikipedia:

Chlorpromazine, marketed as Thorazine, was first synthesized on December 11, 1951. It was the first drug developed with specific antipsychotic action and would serve as the prototype for the phenothiazine class of drugs, which comprises several other agents. The introduction of chlorpromazine during the 1950s has been described as the single greatest advance in the history of psychiatric care, improving the prognosis of people in psychiatric hospitals. Chlorpromazine is on the World Health Organization's List of Essential Medicines, a list of the most important medications needed in a basic health system.

Everything in our lives carries relative risks: hoped-for benefits versus the risk of undesirable repercussions. How would you react to some of the listed caveats in evaluating your use of Thorazine? These things include sedation and the failure of the drug to work (and the prospect of relapse) when you tapered it off to zero; weight gain; decreased blood pressure with dizziness, liver irritation with jaundice (bile that causes the skin and whites of the eyeballs to yellow), and liver failure; and Parkinsonism, which produces symptoms such as tremor, hesitancy of movement, decreased facial expression, and even death. If these don't give you pause, how about the fact that Thorazine can cause a condition called tardive dyskinesia, which manifests as involuntary movements? "Tardive" means delayed, and "dyskinesia" means abnormal movements such as facial grimacing, finger movement, jaw swinging, repetitive chewing, and tongue thrusting, all of which are also possible in Parkinsonism.

The term "caregiver" hadn't been popularized in the 1950s, but that was exactly the role I was handed. I never entertained a thought about walking away from seeing my wife recover from this acute medical challenge. I took my marriage vows seriously, as I did the oaths to my chosen mistress, medicine. *I'm a doctor, damn it*, I told myself; *I'll get her through this.*

I would periodically have to entertain fleeting thoughts about our future. We had planned to have several children. She most assuredly would be on medications for the rest of her life. Could we safely create a child? I knew bipolarism carried a genetic component, and there was no testing for that. I would never want to chance passing bipolarism on to children. I would have no problem adopting children, but how about Joan? Would she be able to teach, raise children, and interact socially? And what type of professional career could I handle while taking care of Joan at the same time? Then there was the $64,000 question: What about me—the real me? I tried not to dwell on that thought, nor did I discuss it with anyone. Here I am half a century later still learning how to share thoughts that never leave me, emotions that paralyze the senses, and silent cries for help. It's called learning to live with reality. While support, perseverance, and that always-welcome touch of luck have made it more livable, I kid you not, I still sometimes entertain the thought of escaping everything and disappearing into another life.

As a first-generation American and a Jewish minority exposed to overt and punishing bullying, bias, and prejudice, I developed defense mechanisms early on in my life. I persevered and succeeded. But what about now? How would I handle this bombshell? This was a life-altering challenge to our marriage vow, "Till death do us part."

Yes, in today's advice to caregivers, we address guilty feelings, responsibilities, asking for help, taking care of yourself, and knowing your limitations. No such world existed in the 1960s; a caregiver essentially walked alone through a valley of trip wires. Then, as now, if you didn't have financial resources, family support, and a ton of luck, you and your significant other succumbed to tragic endings such as divorce, abandonment, or suicide. I've seen it all through more than half a century of personal experience in providing health care for others. Dealing with ever-present challenges and developing sensitivities have made me a better physician and a more resilient person, but in all honesty I would have preferred some other process and a different educational experience.

To this day, in the twenty-first century, many unanswered questions are still not being pursued. The main reason, unfortunately, is the absence of financial incentive, which is the engine that drives the bulk of our research. Funding basic research is left to taxpayer-supported institutions such as the National Institutes of Health (NIH), privately motivated philanthropy, or economically driven product development.

After approximately five weeks at Walter Reed hospital in 1959 I received a call from Joan's psychiatrist at Walter Reed Hospital. He thought she could try a day of freedom in the DC area. She was still on a sizeable dose of Thorazine but was able to communicate and function reasonably well. We agreed on a Sunday. Walter Reed provided hotel-like rooms in a nearby building. Active service members paid nothing, and relatives paid a nominal fee. Joan's mother and my mother had both let me know early on in her hospitalization that they wanted to take a train from New York City and to be with me when Joan was allowed visitors. While they both meant well, I saw no need for their support and even felt that their presence might be counterproductive. I would have preferred that they stay in New York. My perception of Joan's mother was that she was a passive-dependent person who denied that her husband and son were struggling to cope with their bipolar issues. She expected them to take care of her. Joan's brother had the continuous task of doing family errands and overseeing his father's role as a traveling salesman who sold advertising novelties such as key chains, rain bonnets, hair brushes and of course imprinted t-shirts. It took a toll on his marriage and his work as an accountant. I wondered why she was coming down.

Similarly, I saw no benefit in my mother coming down. Obviously, I was not in a forgiving nor understanding mood. Maybe, in a way, I was blaming Joan's mother for my predicament; I also didn't relish the thought of my mother making an inappropriate comment about my not having done a better job in selecting a mate. Catskill Mountain resort humor—humor from what was referred to as the Borscht Belt—always referred to a Jewish mother being snobbish about whom her doctor son married. It happened to be humor that was based in fact. My mother and mother-in-law did come down, and Joan seemed to enjoy seeing them and hearing the reassurances they offered that she was, and would be, fine.

When Joan rejoined me at Fort Detrick, my colleagues were exemplary in never asking us questions about her absence or treating her differently from other spouses. It was obvious to me that her "affect" (mood) was blunted; she was not the usual bubbly person I was accustomed to. Her interest or ability to initiate intimacy was nonexistent. She was aware of the change and she would occasionally remark: "I don't like the *blah feeling* my medicine causes. I prefer being more hyper."

I tried newer medications as they came on the market. All seemed to blunt affect, decrease libido, and cause other side effects such as constipation, dry mouth, and a lowered tolerance for alcohol. It seemed like she flirted with periodic depressive moods followed by an upswing to hypomania: never over the line in either direction, but coming close enough to get my attention. It seemed to occur more commonly in the spring and fall. The medical literature has noted similar observations, including the positive influences of sunlight as opposed to cloudy, overcast days. We hired live-in help with the kids and took periodic vacations both with and without the children. As far as our world knew, we were the ideal young, successful couple living the American Dream. I felt like I was sitting atop a volcano that rumbled enough to continuously remind me of its awesome, restless power. Fortunately, I was too busy and focused on solving medical problems for others, as well as family challenges, to think much about my long hours of perpetual motion against a backdrop of Joan's delicate mood status.

I've said before that luck has played a significant role in my life. The history of lithium therapy is a good example. Yes, this is the same element that is used in our very popular lithium ion batteries that power cars, airplanes, and numerous electronic devices. It is a naturally occurring, silver-white, very light metal that is found in the earth. Several physicians in several countries during the 1800s used it for various clinical conditions, including what was known as "mood stabilization." Its early effective use to mitigate or prevent depressive illness was largely ignored until an Australian physician named Dr. John Cade reintroduced lithium to psychiatry for mania in 1949. I have read that it wasn't until 1970, however, that the United States became the fiftieth country in the world to admit lithium to the marketplace. I used it for my wife in the late 1960s. In fact, as far as I know, I was the first physician to use it in Westchester County.

The nearest psychiatrist for the city of Peekskill had his main office about twenty-five miles to the south of us (toward New York City), in the Croton-on-Hudson area. He also had a part-time office in Peekskill. I asked him if he would put Joan on lithium. He was not enthusiastic about doing it and quoted the following: "WARN-ING: Lithium toxicity is closely related to serum lithium levels, and can occur at doses close to therapeutic levels. Facilities for prompt and accurate serum lithium determinations should be available before initiating therapy."

Our local hospital could monitor the serum levels of lithium, and as a physician I was as qualified as anyone to give it a try. I saw a remarkable response within two weeks. The brand name, Eska-lith, by Smith, Kline & French pharmaceuticals, was very inexpensive: five dollars for a month's supply of ninety capsules. Joan was very stable with three capsules a day, and the only adverse effect she experienced (after thirty-five to forty years on the medication) was that her thyroid function was knocked out. She easily and effectively went on thyroid-replacement tablets in the late 1980's.

An interesting new patient called my office approximately six weeks after I put Joan on Lithium. He asked if he could come in and talk to me. I set up a time after regular hours. He was my age, married with three children, and his problem was his bipolar wife. He told me he was considering divorce and/or committing his wife to a psychiatric institution if he could get it done and if he could afford it. He purged his frustrations to me in dealing with health-care providers, functioning at work, and trying to explain realities to their children, all with little understanding or help from his in-laws and bewilderment from his parents. I explained that a new medication was available and I outlined the benefits and precautions, to which he replied, "I don't have anything to lose, Doc; let's go for it."

I met his wife, listened to her story, and examined her. She did remarkably well, just like Joan. For me, lithium still remains a first-choice option for treating bipolar disease. The pharmaceutical companies, however, are not pushing it, since the profit margins are miniscule compared to newer—but not necessarily better, and definitely more expensive—medications.

The fact remains that we do not know how lithium really works in moderating bipolar disease, nor do we know what contribution or association it makes toward later cognitive impairment.

It may be a very long time, if ever, that anyone will look for those answers without monetary incentives. At the time, I was given the number of 85 percent effectiveness in treating bipolar patients; I have read recently that it's more like 30 percent. I don't know what is closer to the truth, but if I were faced with treating a bipolar patient, that is the first medication I would try. The second choice would be generic Depakote.

I closed my practice in Peekskill in 1973 and moved to Las Vegas, where I would become medical director for the United States nuclear test program in Nevada. This meant a decided cut in income, but this was offset by a nine-to-five job with many enjoyable challenges. I was forty-three, and Joan was thirty-seven. The children enjoyed growing up in the relatively small city of Las Vegas and went on to become self-sufficient and productive members of society. Joan had a lot to do with their positive maturation by getting very involved with their religious and public schooling and keeping them busy with tennis and other extracurricular activities. She was a good bridge player, skier, real estate agent, and community volunteer. She enjoyed the company of many friends and entertained quite often.

As I've shared many times with patients, families, doctors in training, and at public forums: never ever prejudge an individual's potential, regardless of the diagnosis and attendant challenges. Whether it's Down's syndrome, autism, or stage-four melanoma, all people are individual cases unto themselves, and the miracle of individual achievement can be awesome. My wife's successful personal life as a wife, mother, teacher, and community activist, despite the challenges of dealing with bipolarism, is a testament to the art and science of healing: always proceed with the premise that we can do better if we give it a try.

It was the best of times and the most challenging of times, to paraphrase old man Dickens. I enjoyed the transition from being a solo family doctor who was on call twenty-four hours a day, seven days a week, to a chief corporate medical officer who had what was essentially a nine-to-five, weekend-free job. I easily took to outlining policies and goals and delegating responsibility to a large medical staff. But wearing several hats when interacting with federal and state government officials, scientific laboratories, workers and their families, and the local medical communities took a little extra time. It worked very well until my eighteenth year on the job. The chief manager of the Nevada operations office of the Department of Energy didn't like a memo I wrote and he fired me. I won my case without a lawyer. It's all in my book, *The Obligated Volunteer*, available at CreateSpace.com.

Joan's transition to the wife of a corporate physician in southern Nevada was an extension of our American Dream. She complemented my professional and social interactions. We had friends, status, and positively involved children. Joan did not want anyone to know about her history of bipolarism or about her medications. No one did know: not even the children. It worked, but I never dropped my surveillance, so to speak. I made sure she took her lithium and I carefully watched for any troubling behavioral signs.

I bought the lithium through mail order and, using a false name, I did periodic testing for lithium blood levels. I had no thoughts about dementia, even though Joan's mother and two aunts had developed it in their early eighties. We were a productive family enjoying the fruits of hard work, love, biblical-style ethical roots, and lots of good luck.

It was thirty-three years after moving to Las Vegas that our psychiatrist son in Tucson astutely questioned subtle changes he'd noticed in Joan's responses during routine conversations: changes like getting events out of sequence and not following through with thoughts. I, nor anyone else, noticed these subtle changes. He administered a simple, fifteen-minute word test called the "Mini-Cog." He did not need expensive laboratory tests, psychology profiles, consultations, or sleep or imaging studies such as CAT (also known as CT) scans, MRIs, or PET-CT scans, described in chapter 2. The Mini-Cog is a simple test that can easily be administered by an assistant in any family practitioner's office. It reinforces the basic science and art of medicine: one does a complete history and a physical examination, followed by selective, appropriate testing, and then takes time to use his or her brain to analyze differential diagnostic possibilities and options. Too many physicians, for a variety of reasons (such as time constraints and financial incentives), have forgotten the art and science of medical practice to the detriment of patient care.

"Dad," he said, "I did a Mini-Cog test on Mom, and she does show signs of early cognitive impairment: early dementia of some sort."

"Kevin," I responded, "What are you talking about?"

"I do this for a living, Dad. I'm sure about what I'm saying. As you know, we can do a lot of testing to try to figure out whether it might be Alzheimer's or something else, but most likely we won't find much. We wouldn't have anything to offer for prevention no matter what we might find. I'd say we should do nothing for now, and let's see how it goes."

That's exactly what we did, and within a few years the diagnosis of dementia was proven correct. We will discuss the type of dementia she has, and the use of medications to combat it, in subsequent chapters. I have my ideas, which don't always agree with those of our son or other medical colleagues. Needless to say, I've had to make very difficult decisions about medical testing and consulting. With considerable resolve and compassion, I have had to develop skills to console Joan as her world turned upside down—as did my own. Her dementia diagnosis has actually been very much like a replay of her bipolar diagnosis. It did not appear suddenly as her first manic episode; it was a very subtle onset. However, the options were very limited then with bipolar disease and are very limited now with dementia. The challenges are continue to be endless.

I took away her driver's license and I tried to explain why she couldn't play bridge or tennis. I took over all the family functions such as shopping, cleaning the house, doing the wash, balancing the checkbook, and doing our books for taxes. Fortunately, she accepted my explanations and actions without much pushback. She was aware that "she was having problems," as she occasionally put it. I also knew that she was experiencing moments of fear and anxiety, since she would sometimes reach out to touch me during the night.

"Are you OK?" I would ask.

"Yes, I just wanted to make sure you were there. I love you; good night."

I can't imagine how I would react to moments, fleeting as they may be, in which I felt alone, confused, and totally helpless. I've had two dreams of being intubated and coming out of coronary bypass surgery unable to move or breathe on my own and conscious enough to be aware of my dependence on machines. I will never forget the sheer terror I felt of not being in control.

My conclusion has been that Joan's thoughts are very fleeting. They are rapid, short lived, and all over the place. As a consequence, she does not have time to dwell on anything. I take advantage of this to easily change the subject if she appears to be heading toward confusion and discomfort. Reassurance with smiles, hugs, and kisses is the medicine that always works best. Each case has its own puzzle; some are more difficult than others. With Joan, the thought that keeps recurring to me is the realization that her condition is progressive. We can no longer share memories as we once did, nor can we share the joy of seeing our children and grandchildren thrive; that which we helped create, nurture, and mature. If people ask me, "How are things going?" I can only respond with, "Could be worse." It's not really consoling; it's cold reality.

Anyone with a biology background understands that we are born with genetic potential. That potential is passed from generation to generation, and sometimes it gets damaged, for good or for bad, and sometimes it happens with no consequences. The idea is to discover which specific genetic material affects which disease process so that we can then see if we can block or modify the expression of that genetic material. We are making great progress in many areas, but we still have huge gaps in our knowledge. Unfortunately, as with everything else, unethical entrepreneurs have multiplied like cockroaches in a cookie jar when it comes to offering inexpensive and useless testing for genetic profiles or too-good-to-believe panaceas for improving memory, promoting superhuman vigor, and thwarting the aging process. Many of us find comfort in varying degrees and types of faith and hope, but we have to be realistically disciplined to separate the honest and dedicated people who are looking for answers from those who are only looking to separate people from their assets.

Here's a quote that deserves continual presence, from *Vegas HealthCare Quarterly*, 2015, Volume 8: "Intervention and Education Are Key to Helping Mental Illness," by Amanda Llewellyn.

> The stigma of mental illness is a paradox; it's all around us but creates a blanket of anonymity that keeps sufferers unseen

and often untreated for months, years, decades or sometimes a lifetime. Although people suffering from mental illness are more likely to seek help today than they were ten years ago, this stigma often shames many into silence.

If you think we have improved care in mental-health medicine, view the first segment of TV's *60 Minutes*, from August 2, 2015. It may be shocking to you; it's old news to me. I will address this true story later in the book. It clearly shines a light on society's failure to put mental-health research and care at the top of our priority to-do list.

CHAPTER I

UNDERSTANDING WORDS

Iatrogenic = Doctor caused

Cognition = Equivalent to thinking

Recent research suggests that medication, while sometimes help-ful, may cause even greater problems than it solves because of side effects such as worsened cognition and drowsiness. It is hard to admit that some medical professionals are guilty of not learn-ing what is available and what is generally considered standard knowledge and principles of medical practice. If health-care pro-viders do not admit to those shortcomings, then their patients and their patients' lawyers will continue to escalate malpractice claims. The general populace also have to recognize that health-care professionals do not know all there is to know. We do make honest mistakes that only come to light when we learn something new: something that seems obvious in the present but was totally off the radar when the diagnosis, medication, or procedure was first made and applied. Medicine is not an exact science. For example, prefrontal lobotomies, which I will address later, are surgical procedures that are intended to destroy brain tissue for "unruly" mental patients. At one time the procedure was done in good faith, but it became totally unacceptable starting in the mid-twentieth century when drugs like rauwolfia and the afore-mentioned chlorpromazine were discovered to better manage the behavioral changes that result from serious mental illness.

We know that certain naturally occurring risks of birth defects exist that are beyond the obstetrician's knowledge and control; these types of risk are estimated to occur at 2–10 percent of all births. It is understandable to want to blame someone or some-thing when such a tragedy occurs. The mother may even blame herself and initiate postpartum depression, or what is sometimes referred to as an "ambulance-chaser" may seek to create a mer-itless case against a medication and/or a physician. Sometimes there are very legitimate gray areas. It takes objectivity and dis-cipline to try to conduct the right evaluation for the benefit of all involved.

We must hold health-care providers accountable for not adhering to the usual and customary standards of care and we must guard against frivolous and unfounded allegations. The patient must also be held accountable for making informed con-sent, which means gathering and understanding what is being discussed in terms of diagnoses, treatment plans, and options. If the patient is too cognitively impaired, then a guardian, caregiver, or advocate must be designated who has legally documented power of attorney to make medical and financial decisions.

Everything has to be written and legally witnessed. If no read-ily available written documents can be found to use for reference, then a totally preventable mess will most likely happen.

The Difference between Neuroses and Psychoses

Keep in mind that making an accurate assessment of a patient's problem can be very easy or very, very difficult—and everything in between—even with the best-trained and best-equipped providers. It's more difficult with psychiatric patients, since the provider has to rely more on taking careful histories, paying attention to details (subtle as well as overt), and remaining objective. In my opinion, it is an extremely labor-intensive process.

At some point in everyone's life, the question arises: Am I going nuts? (Or is someone else going nuts?) If you ask that question, you very well may be exhibiting neurotic behavior (neuroses or psychoneuroses) such as some degree of anxiety, obsessive-compulsive fixation, or a paralyzing fear of something like flying or leaving the house (i.e., a phobia). By asking the question, you indicate that you are still in contact with reality, which by definition means that you are *not* going crazy (i.e., becoming psychotic). You are trying to deal with exaggerated forms of normal thinking, behavior, and feeling. This is primarily acquired, may seriously hamper your normal daily activities, and can and should be treated if it rises to the level of interfering with your day-to-day life. Medications may help the patient to become more receptive and pliable to an understanding of (and desensitization to) his or her condition. Contrary to what some people believe, more serious mental illnesses, such as schizophrenia or manic depression (i.e., psychosis), do *not* develop from anxiety states.

Psychoses, on the other hand, refers to a serious condition in which the patient has lost contact with reality. Patients cannot control impulses or make decisions; they may have insomnia or delusions, which may cause them to hear voices; they may experience appetite loss; and they may lack cognition and coherent speech. Psychoses are neurologic diseases with genetic components that are triggered by many different stressors; positive family histories may often be found. Psychotic behavior may also arise from traumatic brain injury, as may occur from auto accidents, on the battlefield, or from playing sports.

Genetics plays no direct role in brain injury cases. Psychotic episodes may wax and wane and they may become more frequent or last longer than they once did. The patient will eventually require more care. I know of no cure for psychoses: only various approaches to management. Two of the most common psychoses are schizophrenia and bipolar disease. The deterioration in these diseases is linked to changes in brain structure and interaction with chemicals that are produced within the brain and/or other parts of the body. Research is ultimately aimed at prevention, but in that regard we have nothing to offer for now except, perhaps, genetic counseling. We do have several options for managing function, using medications and cognitive behavior therapy (CBT). CBT is very labor intensive and costly, however, and it is very difficult to find and/or train enough people to fill the need for its administration. Making an accurate diagnosis in psychiatry is particularly difficult, because some mental conditions have no specific markers within laboratory or imaging studies. They rely heavily on clinical signs and symptoms that may be shared by several different disease states.

Funding for research and development does not adequately address these clinical challenges, since funding comes from three main areas: health-care industries driven by financial motives, individual and group philanthropists, and government grants and subsidies. The last two areas of funding are also driven by special interests. Many of the federal laws have perfectly good intentions, such as Medicare disability support, regardless of age, for those who are truly disabled. But as the journalist Catherine Crier pointed out in her 2002 book *The Case Against Lawyers*, once the legislation leaves Congress, bureaucrats apply their own interpretations for implementation and oversight. Rarely are the originators of the legislation involved in following up to ensure application as they originally intended.

4

A very explicit example of this was presented on *60 Minutes* by the then senator from Oklahoma, Thomas Coburn, MD. He showed a town where over 50 percent of the population was on fraudulent Medicare disability payments. The head of this scheme was a lawyer who openly advertised a 100 percent success rate in Medicare disability claims. That in itself raises the red flag of fraud and abuse. As Senator Coburn explained, applicants came to the lawyer's office, where the lawyer's staff filled out the paperwork from one of the many generic templates they had—papers that had nothing to do with the claimants' real histories or physical exams (neither of which was ever done). The staff then had the physicians on their payroll sign the fraudulent applications, which then went on to a federal judge (who was also on the payroll).

This kind of Medicare fraud and abuse, according to Senator Coburn, cost around $115 billion per year, and he predicted that the Medicare disability trust fund would be out of money by 2016. Add that to the annual losses of Medicare/Medicaid of another $282 billion per year (as stated by the United Health Insurance Company), and it's obvious that those current practices are unsustainable. To clarify, Medicare is a federal program that is aimed at helping people aged sixty-five and older with basic medical coverage; those who are totally disabled from working, regardless of age; and Title V–dependent children. Title V Maternal and Child Health Services Block Grant Program is the Nation's oldest federal-state partnership. It's aim is to improve the health and well-being of women, particularly mothers, and children. Medicaid, which is administered by the states and is partially subsidized by federal funds, is aimed at helping the poor. Both programs suffer from rampant, glaring fraud and abuse.

Dementia: The Big Kahuna

The Mayo Clinic's website titled *Patient Care and Health Information* has the best definition I've seen: "Dementia isn't a specific disease. Instead, dementia describes a group of symptoms affecting memory, thinking and social abilities severely enough to interfere with daily functioning."

The key word is *symptoms*. In other words, the labels we give to the many causes of dementia are based on observation and assumptions. We really have very little understanding of the underlying causes, and that means that we cannot, at this time, prevent or treat the conditions we talk about. Yes, we have medications, physical therapy, and cognitive interactions to help manage the symptoms, and some pharmaceutical companies claim that their medications *may* slow the progression of the symptoms. I have professional and personal reasons to doubt those claims, however, and I bristle at the egregious costs for their products.

I have similar problems with the supplement and additive industry: the so-called health food and vitamin industry. This industry is usually coupled with alternative medicine, and is not subject to Federal Drug Administration (FDA) oversight and compliance. That multibillion dollar industry fleeces the gullible public every minute of the day. One very recent example claims in slick television ads that a newly discovered protein in jellyfish, according to their researchers (unnamed, of course), has been shown to improve memory function as people age. The next thing, I expect, will be smoothies, omelets, and pastries with not only the miraculous jellyfish protein, but maybe a little Colorado cannabis to boot. That combination will be guaranteed to get your mind distracted from thinking about your real problems. Back to the Mayo Clinic:

> Dementia indicates problems with at least two brain functions, such as memory loss and impaired judgment or language, and the inability to perform daily activities such as paying bills or becoming lost while driving.
>
> Though memory loss generally occurs in dementia, memory loss alone doesn't mean you have dementia. There is a certain extent of memory loss that is a normal part of aging. ["Age appropriate" is a good term for this.]

> Many causes of dementia symptoms exist. *Alzheimer's disease* [emphasis added] is the most common cause of a progressive dementia. Some causes of dementia may be reversible.

I disagree with the statement that Alzheimer's disease is the "most common cause of a progressive dementia." It certainly has had the lion's share of media attention, though. But the old saying that "statistics lie, and liars love statistics" is probably true. When we give a name to a disease, that action may rest solely on the disease's clinical signs and symptoms; it may also correlate with laboratory and imaging tests or tests conducted after death, with findings derived from just looking at body parts (gross anatomy) or under the microscope (microscopic anatomy). These days, scientists are attempting more and more to link the disease with genetic markers.

Dr. Aloysius "Alois" Alzheimer (1864–1915) observed that some of his patients had acted with similar psychologic signs and symptoms, such as remembering things in the past but not recently, or that they had lost their ability to recognize family members and friends. When he examined their brains after death, he found their nerve connections to be tangled. Today, when we think we are so smart with our new and extremely expensive imaging systems (CT scans, PET-CT scans, and MRIs, described in the next chapter), we also look for amyloid plaques and tau protein as possibly being linked to Alzheimer's disease. Amyloid and tau protein are abnormal proteins—chemicals, if you like. Not all researchers agree on pursuing that line of investigation; indeed, at this point we have no clue about how or why the amyloid or tau proteins appear. To take it a few steps further, we know that some people will have tau or amyloid and never develop Alzheimer's, while some, of course, develop Alzheimer's without ever having markers like tau or amyloid *or* the tangles that Dr. Alzheimer originally described. In other words, the diagnosis of Alzheimer's while the patient is alive is far from conclusive. It is very well accepted among researchers and physicians that at least 30 percent of patients who are clinically diagnosed as having Alzheimer's prove to have had the wrong diagnosis if they receive an autopsy examination.

So how do we decide if we or our loved ones have dementia versus normal age-related forgetfulness? Many times patients and their significant others ignore the issue until it becomes a problem with their daily activities, such as wandering off and getting lost or perhaps even skipping daily hygiene routines to the point of resembling a homeless person. The main point is not to dwell on labels. Physicians (including me) mainly treat behavioral symptoms that interfere with daily living activities. We encourage healthy lifestyles such as quitting (or not starting) smoking, having a good diet, getting plenty of exercise, and engaging in societal interaction; we also correct for comorbid conditions such as diabetes, obesity, elevated blood pressure, and unhealthy cholesterol profiles.

If you are the caregiver-advocate for the patient, and you are lucky, you may find a well-qualified physician who will take the time and effort required to properly assess the patient. The process is very straightforward. It entails taking a detailed history, doing a physical examination, administering one or more fifteen- to twenty-five-minute word tests, and ordering a routine set of laboratory examinations. These steps should provide a working diagnosis with a plan of action, all of which has to be discussed with, and understood by, both the advocate/caregiver and the patient, if he or she is still cognizant enough to comprehend. As stated, medications at this point in time are almost exclusively aimed at managing symptoms. No cures currently exist, and any claims that the process can be slowed carry the caveat, *maybe*. I do not support the use of Aricept (donepezil) or Namenda (memantine HCL) and I bristle at the pharmaceutical companies' brazen practices of slightly altering their formulations strictly for the purpose of extending patent rights, thus leading to even higher medication charges. Pay very close attention to side effects. Do the medical risks and adverse drug and chemical interactions really justify using the medications?

Here are some of the severe signs, symptoms, and diagnostic labels we assign to various forms of dementia, i.e., the loss of one's ability to think and connect with the environment: difficulty processing information; may have long-term memory loss, short-term memory loss, or both; may be unable to avoid disorientation with respect to time, place, or person; may become agitated or withdrawn or go through cycles with both mood states; or may lose the ability to recognize familiar people. Each case is different, and each person may exhibit different groups of symptoms at different times and show different rates of deteriorating progression. Many succumb to strokes or heart attacks that may result from falls, malnutrition, infection, other underlying diseases, or surgical procedures followed by clots or bleeding. We are, after all, attempting to manage life's age-related challenges. With dementias, I guarantee encounters with some sadness, some serenity, and lots of acceptance. There are choices that can be made to lessen the load, but they will not be handed to you on a plate.

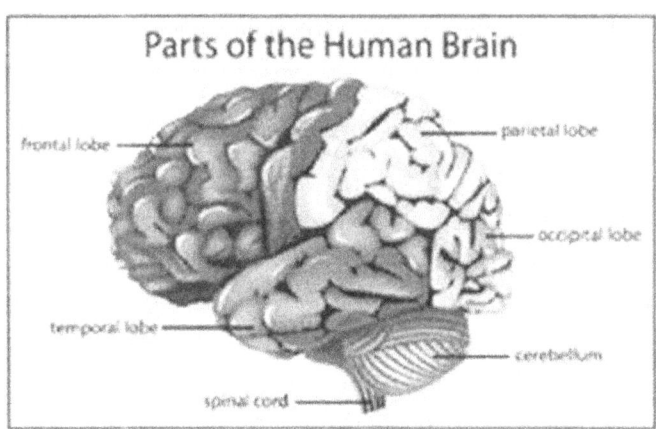

I am a fairly quick learner, but to really understand and retain concepts and information, I usually have to repeat, consider, review again, and maybe do it again a few more times. For this reason, I'll comment on the side view of the brain (above), shown with the protective bony skull removed. The front is to the left and is appropriately named the *frontal lobe* (behind your forehead); the *temporal lobes* are roughly behind each ear; the *parietal lobe* is roughly above the temporal lobes; the *occipital lobe* is at the back of your head and is where your sight is processed; the *cerebellum* is found at the base of the brain and, among other things, controls balance; and the *spinal cord* carries the connections to the entire body for sensory and motor (muscular) function. If you think of the brain as a melon, the rind or peel is the outer shell. With the brain, the outer shell is called the *cortex*, also referred to as the gray matter of the brain. I will refer to this visual portrayal of the brain as we go through different forms of dementia. Once again, from the Mayo Clinic:

> Dementia is not a specific disease. It is a descriptive term for a collection of symptoms that can be caused by a number of disorders that affect the brain. People with dementia have significantly impaired intellectual functioning that interferes with normal activities and relationships. They also lose their ability to solve problems and maintain emotional control and they may experience personality changes.

When talking about the different kinds of dementia, we can do so by referring to the parts of the brain that cause the abnormal behavior, such as *cortical dementia* (coming from the outer surface or gray matter) or *subcortical* (coming from the deeper regions of the brain). We may also characterize the dementia by timeline or by degree of severity, such as *progressive/stationary* or *mild, moderate*, or *advanced*. We may add a term that describes what we think is the etiology (cause), such as *primary dementia*, meaning that it comes from direct dysfunction within the brain tissue; *secondary dementia* would mean that it had been caused by another disease process, such as injury or a chemical or physical cause. So for example, after doing the history and physical exam and the laboratory tests, the physician might make a working diagnosis of fronto-temporal dementia with moderate cognitive impairment secondary to small strokes (circulatory dysfunction).

The physician has the obligation to ensure that the caregiver/ advocate (and patient, if applicable) understands that the diagnoses is a work in progress that is subject to reexamination as he or she tries to manage the patient. It is helpful for the physician to use diagrams and descriptive comparisons to explain how and why the working diagnosis was established.

The next question is inevitable: What caused the dementia, and what can we do to avoid, treat, or manage the various conditions? *Advancing age* carries risk. *Genetics* (family history) may point to any inherited predispositions, which in turn brings up genetic counseling and any factors to avoid that might be likely to trigger unwanted disease processes. If you and your spouse had bilateral family histories of type I diabetes, bipolar disease, Down's syndrome, early onset Parkinsonism, or Alzheimer's, would you adopt children rather than risk creating a family with a significant risk of life-altering functions? I'm not suggesting selective reproduction for a "super race"; I am suggesting difficult considerations to bear in mind based on sound science in order to minimize the risk of serious genetic outcomes.

CHAPTER II

A FEW FACES OF DEMENTIA

According to the Alzheimer's Association, frontotemporal dementia (FTD) is "a group of disorders caused by progressive nerve cell degeneration in the brain's frontal lobes (the areas behind your forehead) or its temporal lobes (the regions behind your ears)."

Keep in mind that when the word *may* is used, it really means that we don't know for sure. The speculation about the cause or treatment of a medical condition may be based on good research and objective reasoning, or, in the case of selling worthless concoctions, it may be pure horse manure aimed at personal gain. The only known risk factor for FTD is a family history of the disease, as scientists have found several genes linked to FTD and have identified several abnormal protein deposits within the brain cells in patients associated with FTD. Exactly how these abnormalities foul things up, however, and why they affect the frontal and temporal lobes (as opposed to some other part of the brain), remain unknown.

My wife and I have lived in a Del Webb retirement community (one of the leading builders of such communities) for quite some time. There are roughly eight thousand homes in the development; when it comes to senior profiles, if you can't find a particular eccentricity in this very diverse cross section of people over fifty-five, then it may not exist. We have everything from "senior moments" of no great consequence to very serious disconnects. Some have nicknamed this place "God's waiting room." I estimate that approximately 5 percent take advantage of the many clubs, recreational facilities, and community-sponsored gatherings the place has to offer.

My wife was an avid bridge player, and one of the early signs that clouds were forming in her thought processes came with the realization that she could no longer play. Her bridge club partners didn't want to hurt our feelings by saying anything to either of us. They just made it difficult for her to find a partner. People frequently think that avoidance or silence is preferable to plain honesty. I finally called and told the head of the club that it would have been better if they had simply told me so that I could then explain it to Joan myself. It definitely hurt, but putting this episode behind us was far better than letting things fester.

By this time Joan was also displaying problems with managing the checking account, working in the kitchen, losing her sense of direction, reading books, and watching television. She also showed a somewhat intriguing loss of smell, which is another apocalyptic horse (so to speak) that rides along with FTD.

One of the saddest moments came while we were watching TV—at least I was watching the program. Joan's eyes were on the screen, but her personal, biologic computer, as usual, was elsewhere. She turned toward me and asked: "Would you have married me if you had known all the problems I would have?"

I licked my lips and swallowed, trying not to show my instant disbelief. It was as if she had read my thoughts at some point in our marriage, and now this thinking had managed to get out. I had often asked myself that question, but I never really came up with an answer. I fleetingly thought about the question during our second year of marriage, when Joan had her first bipolar manic episode. Joan had never asked that question in over a half century of marriage, and I sometimes wondered if she understood the extra effort I thought I was putting in to make things work. FTD does remove inhibitions and impulse control, as well as decision making. With her advancing loss of brain cells, she had now asked a $64,000 question. I didn't want to hurt her feelings and needed a moment to phrase my response. Maybe that's a sign of true love—who knows? "What do you mean, hon?" I asked.

"I know I'm not right," she responded.

I looked into her eyes and gave her the only answer I've been giving myself for all of our married years; it never has been a yes or no answer. "When we got married, we never thought about cloudy, rainy days: only sunshine and roses. Well, we've had some great times, some good times, and some bumps in the road. I, as a doctor, am well aware that life is never smooth, but I think we've been luckier than a lot of others. We have great kids and grandkids, and in many respects they're surpassing what we've accomplished for themselves and their communities. We have great memories and we are still here with each other. The bottom line is that I have gratitude for all the good we had and did."

She smiled, took my hand, and remained staring into my eyes: "I love you!" She closed her eyes and leaned back in her recliner. "I think I'll go upstairs and take a nap."

We don't have an upstairs, and it was after 8:00 p.m. She was going to bed. This was the first time in many years that we had taken time to really connect. It was a short two to three moments in an unlikely setting, but for once I knew that she appreciated my contributions to our marriage. Her look and tone of voice reaffirmed my reasons to be her soul mate "till death do us part." She slept very well that night, and so did I.

One of the fortuitous benefits of FTD is that a patient usually is not able to focus or dwell on a thought for very long; as a result, they don't get very upset by things in general, and inconsequential things that might have become an issue in the past no longer create a challenge. As an example, our daughter once remarked early in Joan's transition: "You know, Mom is much more easygoing and more accommodating than before she had the problems she now has."

Yes, just think how more devastating it might be if Joan dwelled on the fact that she was losing her ability to make decisions, play bridge, remember faces, and not get lost. In general, people with bipolar disease and dementias may show little deep emotion, because their minds are wandering or racing in many different directions. Someone may say to her partner, "I love you," for example, and in the next instant say, "I'm going to play tennis; see you" and disappear. It's more like interacting with a programmed robot. If this occurs, do not expect the person to change. It's not that this person doesn't really love her spouse; she most likely does. She just doesn't have time to slow her brain for warm, fuzzy moments. If you are lucky to have such moments, savor them, but don't expect repeats.

A person who is experiencing dementia will get deeper into his own world. That presents additional challenges to the caregiver. The patient can't help what he says or does. Although no one can change what's going on in his brain, caregivers *can* learn to manage the dementia, such as changing the subject, distracting the person with a photo, or humming a familiar tune. You, as a caregiver, will get nowhere with arguing and raising your blood pressure: that would not be productive for either of you.

I've given you a personal glimpse into my wife's FTD journey. What were some of the medical indicators? Her first MRI in 2009 had a suggestive clue. The radiology report read: "Mild to moderate atrophy of the frontal cortex" [that outer part of the front brain we discussed earlier]. This may be part of normal aging. Clinical correlation is advised."

Indeed, many people who have an MRI of the brain for whatever reason may show some degree of cortical atrophy (i.e., shrinkage) and never show any form of dementia. I have not found any acceptable explanation for this. In my clinical correlation of the MRI report, I agreed then (and still do today) that FTD was exactly what Joan was dealing with, even though other professionals want to repeat the thousands of dollars' worth of imaging and laboratory tests we've had done and prescribe worthless and very expensive medications. For me, she has clinical symptoms that are consistent with fronto-temporal dementia; while there are no effective, definitive treatment options for this condition, certain approaches may help manage her condition better than simply doing nothing.

I enrolled Joan in the Banner Research Brain Bank program in Sun City, Arizona. It is open and free to residents who have lived in Arizona for six months or more. I have included this program in a reference list at the end of my book. The program won't help her, but it will provide valuable information for our family and others. I'm almost certain it will confirm FTD due to failure of the small blood vessels that nourish that part of the brain. Maybe we will eventually get better at understanding, preventing, and managing the nourishment failure process.

Incidentally, MRI stands for magnetic resonance imaging. It's a wonderful invention that uses magnets and computers to create the image and it does not in any way expose the patient to ionizing radiation as would a computerized tomography (CT) scan—also more formally known as a computerized axial tomography (CAT) scan—or a positron emission tomography–computed tomography (PET-CT) scan. Both of those valuable tools are shockingly overused in the pursuit of generating huge profits. Unnecessary CT exams *do* cause significant exposure to ionizing radiation, which in turn can damage human tissue to the point of causing cancer. Prior to ordering any laboratory test, the physician should have conducted a careful history and physical examination; only then should he or she decide on testing, keeping in mind the risks and costs versus the benefit of what is being ordered. In other words, the doctor, patient, or caregiver/advocate should discuss specific value for ordering any test; for instance, what will the physician hope to gain with the test results? When a physician is asked to justify or clarify the diagnosis, asked what other possible diagnosis it might be, or asked what other treatment options are available, too many will angrily respond with something like, "Who are you to tell me how to practice medicine?"

No one is telling anyone how to practice, as long as what the physician is recommending is within legal rules and regulations and is within established and accepted ethical and moral guidelines.

This is very important: if the physician can't take the time to adequately share the what, where, why, and how of the case, then someone else needs to be medically in charge. The art and practice of medicine is a continuous learning process. People who call themselves physicians without being open to transparency are not worthy of inclusion in one of our noblest endeavors: the art and practice of healing.

To summarize what we've gone over so far in this chapter: even if you don't have medical training, your doctor should discuss and answer questions. The Internet can be your research arena. Ask (and continue to ask) questions until you clearly understand the what, where, how, and why of your medical team's thinking.

Again according to the Alzheimer's Association, "The cell damage associated with frontotemporal dementia (FTD) leads to tissue shrinkage (atrophy) and reduced function in the brain's frontal and temporal lobes which control planning and judgment, emotions, speaking and understanding speech and certain types of movement." There are many theories about what causes the cell damage. One cause does show up very often in autopsies by qualified neuropathologists: namely, microvascular shrinkage. In other words, the small blood vessels that supply those parts of the brain stop delivering nutrients and removing waste. Cells die, just as plants and trees in your garden will die if you live in the desert and you stop watering them. We know in general terms what may adversely affect healthy blood vessels: family history or genetic predisposition, diet, exercise, smoking, lifestyle-risk behaviors, and work environments. Specific profiles such as diabetes, high blood pressure, and bad cholesterol patterns can be treated. We still need to learn a lot more, however. The sad part is that the little we do know about possibly mitigating or eliminating brain cell death (namely, by living healthy lifestyles) is not readily accepted by the public. Too many people are just like the unacceptable physician who says, "Don't tell me what to do." Many just want a simple pill to cover the indulgences and to have someone else pay for it. Entrepreneurs are standing by to knowingly promote unproven "remedies" that could also add risk to life itself, such as putting amphetamines and valium into over-the-counter, unregulated health foods and supplements. Many cases of both intentional and unintentional food and supplement adulterations can be found in the occupational medical literature.

My wife has shown just about all of the reduced-function symptoms of FTD, with the most recent being the aphasias: speaking and understanding. The symptoms come and go for minutes, hours, or days, but they will eventually progress in frequency of occurrence and duration. Some people still refer to FTD as Pick's disease, after a physician named Arnold Pick (1851–1924) who first described in 1892 a patient with distinct symptoms that affected language, such as the ability to comprehend and/or express the patient's thoughts.

Symptoms of FTD are grouped into three main categories, depending on which areas of the frontal and temporal areas of the brain are affected. The symptoms may overlap and show variations in both appearance and duration. It's not necessary to go into all the terminology here. It is also not necessary to become a neurologist, a medical specialist in brain and nerve anatomy and function. What *is* important is to have a general understanding of what is being said and what we really know in terms of managing the challenges.

It was an amusing moment when I heard a politician repeat an old phrase as he was campaigning for president of the United States: *I say what I mean and I mean what I say*. I didn't know if he was genuine or if perhaps he was covering his rear. My wife, however, cannot claim to be able to truthfully use that phrase. One could refer to some of her more random statements as gibberish. At times I think I know what she is really trying to say. No matter; I always smile and agree with whatever comes out, and she will usually smile back and move on to whatever else appears on her mental screen. She is at least fortunate that her jumbled understanding and expression does not seem to bother her, as it does with people who have a stuttering problem. Stutterers understand what they want to say but have trouble getting it out. They do not have my wife's FTD with its perverse blessing (if you will) of not being bothered by her disabilities. At least it appears that way to me. The stutterer knows he may never entirely get rid of his problem, which is an embarrassment that will affect every facet of his life. Dwell on that comparison for a few moments, and you will understand my reply to the ever-present question: "Hi Doc, how're you doing today?"

I might smile, frown, or pucker my lips before responding: "It could be worse." I take a cue from my wife and quickly move on to other thoughts, activities, and sublimations. Her erratic responses are involuntary; my responses are deliberately learned and reinforced.

Repetition is good for learning. Let me quote one more summary, again from the Alzheimer's Association:

There is no single test—or any combination of tests—that can conclusively diagnose frontotemporal dementia. FTD is a clinical diagnosis representing a doctor's best professional judgment about the reason(s) for a person's symptoms. Magnetic resonance imaging (MRI) often plays a key role in diagnosis because it can detect shrinkage in the brain's frontal and temporal lobes, which is a hallmark of FTD. In some cases it may be hard to distinguish FTD from Alzheimer's disease.

Note: brain shrinkage (atrophy) may be seen in routine MRIs that are done, for example, after trauma; the patient may have no associated FTD or any other dementia. Clinical correlation by a well-trained, dedicated physician is the best place to start.

As I stated, if the diagnosis is not clear between FTD and Alzheimer's, it realistically makes little difference for clinical management. I have no support for prescribing two widely used and expensive medications (the aforementioned Aricept and Namenda). Furthermore, it's a disgrace that health-care providers inappropriately and deliberately order imaging and other tests solely for the purpose of generating money; this is a direct contribution to the hundreds of *billions* of dollars that are lost annually in Medicare and Medicaid fraud and abuse cases. Let's concentrate on more and better day-care and night-care centers and sound, basic, and coordinated research.

Dr. Alois Alzheimer

In 1901, Dr. Alzheimer had a fifty-one-year-old female patient who exhibited language and memory problems accompanied by disorientation and hallucinations. Her clinical presentation fit the pattern of what, at the time, was called *dementia*. She was rather young for that diagnosis, however, so Dr. Alzheimer labeled her as having *presenile dementia*. She died five years later, and since Dr. Alzheimer had never seen such a case at that age, he performed an autopsy with the permission of the woman's family. He found the evidence that was usually found among older patients with those clinical presentations: marked atrophying of the cortex, the thin outer layer of gray matter previously described in chapter 1. He also noted two abnormal deposits inside and between the nerve cells. The deposits outside the nerve cells are what we call *amyloid plaques* today (mentioned earlier); these plaques are the subject of many researchers' work. Many think that these may hold the key to a better understanding of Alzheimer's-type dementia. The deposits inside the nerve cells, which are sometimes described as looking like a bowl of spaghetti, are called *neurofibrillary tangles*. Others have also documented these deposits in older patients.

Some patients, we now recognize, may have one or both types of deposits and may indeed not show clinical symptoms of any type of dementia when they are autopsied for some other reason. Others may have clinical symptoms that we label Alzheimer's, and when they are autopsied they have neither type of deposit. So here we are roughly one hundred years later with all our technological advances, but we are still in the dark about the how and why. Dr. Alzheimer presented his case of early dementia in 1906 and didn't seek, or expect, his name to be given to a complex disease that he had recognized in a younger-than-usual patient. It was his boss, Dr. Emil Kraepelin (1856–1926), who had put the label on that group of patients, and it stuck.

Dr. Alzheimer was indeed a pioneer in correlating clinical findings with anatomical changes. As stated, it may be difficult clinically to separate FTD and Alzheimer's, but it's a case of going with the preponderance of evidence for one or the other. The main reason for making a correct diagnosis is to better manage the patient and advise others who are affected. We have *no proven, absolute* tools to avoid the two dementias from occurring, or curing the patient once these dementias appear. Lifestyle changes, diet, or medications have *not* been conclusively shown to do what the promoters say they will. If they were right, we would see clear evidence in declining numbers of dementias, not rising numbers in an aging population. With any luck, we will in the future. Remember, these two dementias do have overlapping presentations, and the physician may have to change the original, working diagnosis, especially if the case proceeds to autopsy. At least 30 percent of the time, a diagnosis of Alzheimer's during a patient's life does *not* match the anatomic findings after death.

Below are a few key differences we look for in deciding on FTD versus Alzheimer's; since there are few absolutes in life, everything carries the caveat "usually."

- **Age at diagnosis**. Alzheimer's is usually diagnosed after seventy years of age; FTD usually appears when patients are in their fifties and sixties.
- **Changes in behavior**. These changes occur more often as the first signs in FTD, such as getting lost, having problems balancing the checkbook, or forgetting how to play cards. Behavioral changes among Alzheimer's patients tend to occur later in the disease's progression.
- **Memory loss**. This is a more prominent symptom in early Alzheimer's; it shows later in FTD. In addition, with Alzheimer's the memory loss is more pronounced when recalling recent events rather than when recalling memories from way back in a patient's life.
- **Hallucinations and delusions**. These are relatively uncommon in FTD, but just the opposite is the case as Alzheimer's progresses.
- **Problems with speech**. While Alzheimer patients may be slow to recall the proper words to use or they may have difficulty remembering names, they don't seem to have the same difficulty in making sense when they speak, understanding what others are saying, reading books, or following what's on television.

- **Problems with spatial orientation**. Getting lost in familiar places is more common among Alzheimer's patients than among FTD patients.

When the diseases reach *end-stages*, they may show symptoms that are indistinguishable from one another, and while autopsy findings may explain some of the clinical signs, symptoms, and overlap, at other times the findings explain nothing. As stated, I have enrolled my wife in the Brain Bank program with Banner Research in Sun City, which is open to all Arizona residents. Consider this program (or one like it), and if you agree in the merits of postmortem examination, I urge all American citizens to find the program closest to your area and make sure that all of the directives and permissions have been prepared. The fact is that we will all die, and by making the necessary arrangements to aid research leading up to and after death, we will hasten our understanding of the disease processes.

Some professionals and patients have trouble accepting facts, and I agree that it may be difficult to do and still provide hope. Without disciplined research and clinical trials, however, we waste money and time and actually do harm by promoting false hope. Some people, from all walks of life, take advantage of the vulnerable in the caregiver world, which is totally unacceptable. As Ronald Reagan famously said, "Trust, but verify."

Treatment and Outcomes in Frontotemporal Disease

"Current FTD treatment focuses on managing symptoms; primarily those affecting behavior. Emerging insights into specific protein abnormalities associated with FTD may identify targets for new treatments aimed at underlying disease processes.

"Antidepressants and antipsychotic drugs are the chief medications used to treat behavioral FTD symptoms. It is very important to note that none of these drugs have been approved by the US Food and Drug Administration (FDA) for use in FTD."

This statement, while true, presents the dilemma of "off-label use," which could indeed invite a lawsuit against a physician. But my wife, with her long personal and family history of bipolar disease, has correctly been treated with antidepressant and antipsychotic medications, and she continues to need them. Documentation is the necessary answer. The physician, if she decides to go off-label, has to clearly document why she is doing it; one example could be that no other options are available for the effective treatment of this patient and the risks versus benefits have been clearly explained to the patient, his or her advocate, and/or other authorized members of the family.

"FTD inevitably gets worse, usually over several years. In advanced FTD, people typically become mute and bedbound. As with other types of dementia, FTD shortens lifespan. Studies suggest that most people with FTD survive an average of six to eight years, but survival can range from two to twenty years."

Alzheimer's Treatments and Outcomes

These treatments and outcomes aren't much different from FTD disease. The FDA has approved two medications for Alzheimer's; the FDA states that they are not cures, but may slow the progression. As stated, I do not accept the pharmaceutical companies' data as convincing. As noted earlier, the two medications' trade names are Namenda and Aricept (or Exelon, which is the patch version made by another company). Behaviors run all over the place when patients use the drugs, running the gamut from withdrawal to over aggression. Slips, trips, and falls are significant and deadly challenges. We do the best we can in our home by removing loose rugs, providing a walker, and making sure areas are well lit. I hope that caregivers do not assume guilt if such tragic events do occur. I, as well as members of my family, were less than a foot from my wife when she lost her balance and fractured her wrist and hip. We could not catch her or lessen the impact of the fall. Health-care professionals should definitely address these feelings of guilt with all family members, and again, *clearly explain and document everything*.

We give labels for other forms of dementia, but we have little (if anything) to offer in terms of prevention or definitive treatment. It's mostly management. Next to Alzheimer's and FTD, a great number of dementias are related to the following problems.

- **Vascular (circulation) problems**. Strokes refer to a sudden blockage or hemorrhage in the brain. Other factors that affect circulation include hardening of the arteries (atherosclerosis), car accidents, sports (professional and recreational), military situations, and environmental toxins.
- **Lewy bodies**, named for their discoverer, Frederic Henry Lewy (1885–1950), can be associated with dementias and movement disorders like Parkinsonism. These bodies refer to abnormal protein deposits in the brain that are only seen with postmortem examination. One cannot definitively include them in a living patient's differential diagnosis, since they do not show up in any imaging screens or laboratory tests. Their significance may be determined at some point in the future.
- **Genetic influence** has been mentioned with FTD (and bipolar disorder); such influence is very clear in **Huntington's disease**, which is (fortunately for most people) a rare hereditary disorder.
- **Mad cow disease (Creutzfeldt-Jakob disease)** is a very rare disease that is believed to be due to *prions*, which fall somewhere between (or perhaps beyond) viruses and bacteria. The disease can also arise through inheritance; it is also possible that it arises from nothing we can explain.
- **Challenges of conception, birth, and development** encompass various conditions that are still difficult to determine in terms of cause, prevention, or treatment; these include conditions such as cerebral palsy and vari-

ous degrees of autism. We know mishaps during birth can be devastating, but serious challenges may also come about with apparently normal prenatal care and delivery.

I have briefly mentioned these last few categories because by my estimate, at least one third of the people in the United States (over one hundred million people) are either directly or indirectly affected by various caregiver dilemmas and challenges. In the following chapters I will try to point out some of the shortfalls that we must address. To some this may sound like an angry tirade by a frustrated professional, husband, and father. Yes, I'm frustrated and angry, but if I don't accept the existence of shortfalls and expose them to the light of day, how can I expect any positive change to occur? We've made huge inroads in public health and are beginning to get a glimpse into the mysteries of immunotherapy and cancer. We must include mental health in our top priorities. It's never easy, and too often the activist with valid intentions becomes the target of angry "push-backers." Put another way, "Please don't kill the messenger."

CHAPTER III

TRANSPARENCY AND ACCOUNTABILITY

I recommend viewing the first thirty-minute segment of the *60 Minutes* episode from August 2, 2015, that I briefly referred to earlier. It clearly exposes an insurance industry practice that is obviously amoral and illegal. If you have experienced this practice, I urge you to write your congressional delegation and demand corrective action.

The case presented involved Anthem Blue Cross and Blue Shield. A mother had a fully paid insurance policy that covered her young bipolar daughter. The daughter displayed behavior that was consistent with an acute manic episode that required life-saving treatment. The mother took her daughter to a hospital emergency room, where she received the appropriate acute care. The ER physician, in accordance with insurance policy requirements, immediately requested written approval for follow-up care; this is customary and usual practice with bipolar patients who are coming off severe manic episodes, since the possibility of such patients harming themselves or others remains very high. It is also standard practice to keep such patients under surveillance and medicated until reasonable stability has been achieved.

Such requests to the insurance company for additional surveillance and treatment are handled by an insurance-company-contracted physician, who then reviews the request and renders approval or disapproval. In this case the doctor in question—nicknamed "Dr. Denial" for his 92 percent denial rate—got forty-five dollars per case and (according to *60 Minutes*) processed about five hundred fifty cases per month, which made him somewhere around $25,000 each month. He used robotic signatures and drew from "copy and paste" generic statements. In other words, if you compared his denial letters, they would sound the same in terms of phrases, form, and, of course, content.

Insurance companies love denials, since they save them money. Neither the insurance company in this case nor the physician agreed to appear on camera. The mother was forced to take her daughter home. The next morning she found her daughter dead from a suicide. If I were on the licensing board of medical examiners for that doctor's state, I would bring that physician up on malpractice charges and accessory to murder. At the very least he would have his license permanently revoked. He knew exactly what he was doing and deliberately ignored usual and customary medical practice based on his personal greed. Because it is also obvious that this was not an isolated case, I would recommend that the insurance company be charged as a coconspirator and forced to pay a very, very high fine. If you were in the jury box, what value would you put on that girl's young life? Why do I mention this case? As you will see, this is the exact same practice that is condoned by Medicare and its designated contractors.

Before I proceed with my wife's case, let me give you a few examples of why I am outraged and frustrated and why I wonder if the good people of this country will ever bring us back to honesty, integrity, and commitment to promises that are made. A copy of my wife's case was sent by registered mail marked Personal in big, bold, black letters; it was also e-mailed (just to be safe) to the newly appointed head of Health and Human Services (HHS), Sylvia Mathews Burwell. During her public appearance in which she accepted President Barack Obama's appointment to the post, she outlined all the good things she was going to do, including working closely with the medical community. I suppose I don't live in the medical community she was referring to, because the only answer I received from her was a form letter that stated how much she appreciated hearing from people in the health-care industry. That was it.

To go back even further, President Obama, when making horse-trading deals with former senators Tom Daschle of South Dakota, Harry Reid of Nevada, and others to get votes for his Affordable Care Act—look it up, it's a matter of public record— he publicly acknowledged that medical practice tort reform was legitimately open for review and action. He said he was directing Kathleen Sibelius, Secretary of HHS, to look into it. The next day, Howard Dean, a physician and former governor of Vermont, was asked about that on the evening news hour. He laughed and responded with something like: Don't hold your breath. Kathleen Sibelius is a former head of the Kansas trial lawyers association; it won't happen.

I may have paraphrased a few words, but the message is accurate; nothing ever did happen. The next day Dean was again asked about his comments on Sibelius looking into medical tort reform. He clearly had a tough time toning his statement down, as his handlers must have directed; I imagine it was like asking the jury to disregard something they have already heard. I suppose he never learned from his presidential campaign outbursts: spilled milk is hard to put back in the bottle. Having lived through all of this infamous and deliberate false rhetoric, you may well ask why I didn't give up with my wife's case. My answer is simple: silence is not an option if you want accountability and hope for positive change.

This is my wife's experience in the medical-rehabilitation-industry that was created and abetted by Medicare. As with many pieces of legislation, the intent may be valid and laudable, but the application lacks oversight and accountability: self-regulation does not work. I suggest again that you read the book *The Case Against Lawyers*, by the aforementioned Catherine Crier, who herself is a lawyer, judge, writer, and TV personality.

A few years back (probably in an election year), our legislators decided to add more perks to Medicare coverage: namely, rehabilitation services in a hospital, a rehabilitation facility, and at home. While the intent was medically valid, the usual lack of professional oversight and accountability has spawned financial bonanzas for entrepreneurs and charlatans in all facets of what is called rehabilitation medicine: physicians, equipment and medical suppliers, physical therapists, and food services, as well as all levels of personnel with a job title of some kind or a description such as medical assistant. Many times these people engage in medical practices that are unnecessary and may even compromise the patient and cause death.

I will point this out in my wife's case. Just about every hospital has added an acute rehabilitation unit. Free-standing rehabilitation facilities (some of which are combined with other levels of care) have similarly sprung up all over the landscape to suck up the cash cow called Medicare. We have group homes, memory care, independent living, assisted living, and skilled nursing. We have entertainers for cognitive enhancement, physical therapists, various levels of psychology assessment and therapy, and pharmaceutical suppliers that (for a fee) will claim to make it easier and more accurate to have them join the party by packaging the medications into foolproof dispensing containers. Nothing escapes the roving eye of American entrepreneurial ingenuity.

I had managed to care for Joan at home for approximately ten years after our psychiatrist son's first confirmation that she had early cognitive dementia. On the tenth year we had gathered at our daughter's home in Scottsdale for the family's Thanksgiving celebration. Two days later, as I've mentioned above, Joan lost her balance, with us standing right next to her, and she fell to the ground and broke her right wrist and right hip. The acute care by the orthopedist and medical physician was excellent, but her transfer to an acute rehabilitation facility (owned by the same general hospital that gave her surgical and medical care) was the beginning of a journey through infamy. I supplied the information requested by the rehab facility, and the transfer was made. A registered nurse (RN) appeared in Joan's room a few hours after her arrival. I volunteered information about Joan's cognitive problems to make sure that they knew that part of her history. The RN pointed to a small blackboard in the room that had her name and position: "Case manager." It also had the name of the physiatrist assigned to Joan; a board-certified MD trained in physical medicine and rehabilitation. The name of the physical therapist who was actually doing the morning and afternoon rehab sessions would be posted daily, with the specific times.

No one ever took a history or did a physical examination. They would have had to ask me more about the patient's medical history, since Joan was cognitively impaired—as I told the RN case manager. I questioned the need for inhalation therapy as well as certain medications. I specifically told the RN and everyone who came into the room that I was Joan's husband, her power of attorney, and a licensed MD. The RN said she would pass the information on to the assigned physician, whom I expected would contact me shortly. She never did. That is pure and simple malpractice. This is what actually happened.

The physical therapists were very good. They took Joan, twice a day, to a large gym-like room, and she followed their rehabilitation protocols. At one end of that room was a glass-enclosed conference room that was clearly visible to everyone in the rehab area. Around the fifth day of Joan's morning workout, I saw three people in the conference room: a man in a white coat, another man in suit and tie, and a woman in a dress. I assumed it might be a staff meeting. I knocked and entered. "Excuse me," I said, "I'm Dr. Kreisler, and my wife is having her morning rehab session." I explained that I had a few questions and passed my card around to each person.

When I offered my card to the woman, she said: "I don't need the card. I know who you are."

"Well, I don't know who you are," I replied.

"I'm your wife's physician. How did you get here?" she asked in a demanding voice.

I took a deep breath, feeling some confusion and disbelief. I felt like giving her a wiseguy answer such as, "I drove here, how else?" Instead, I held my tongue and said the obvious: "Your associated general hospital concluded that my wife was ready for transfer to an acute rehab facility and they indicated their preference for this facility. This facility obviously accepted her, and they apparently assigned you, but you have never attempted to contact me. I don't understand what you are getting at."

"She could have gone directly to a nonacute facility; not here."

"Since I was not consulted or involved, even though I have power of attorney and I am a physician, why don't you ask the medical team who made the decisions and the transfer?" I'm afraid I said this in a rather angry tone.

The man in the white coat decided to comment: "You know, some people don't like to use their own resources…"

I angrily interrupted him: "You don't know me or anything about me. I assume you may be the head psychiatrist here, and as a physician, you ought to know better than to make negative assumptions without empiric evidence. Yes, I know I'm entitled to fourteen days of acute rehab care under Medicare rules. I did not make the transfer, and the physician assigned to my wife has not taken a history, conducted a physical examination, or discussed the comorbid aspects of the case. Consequently I have serious questions about some of the diagnoses and medications on her chart."

I then had a short, heated exchange with the woman when she told me I could just as easily have taken my wife back to Las Vegas for acute and follow-up rehab. How would you react if you were sitting in the jury box? We're talking about an eighty-year-old woman who is cognitively impaired and who is just days past having a hip replaced and a fractured wrist set. To those who are not medically informed, big problems face such patients who are not properly managed, including hip dislocation, which would require more surgery; wound infection and/or pneumonia; and the causing of a clot to the lung or brain. I fantasized about cross-examining such a physician on the witness stand.

The next day I received retribution for my candid exchange. I was notified that I must find another rehab facility within twenty-four hours. I had checked the website of the assigned physician the day of our encounter. She proudly advertised that she had two offices and that she covered eight hospitals. How can one physician do that and still deliver honest, acceptable medical care to her patients? I had already decided to file claims of malpractice when copies of billings came in for that physician and against the codefendant rehab facility. The facility knew what was going on and had aided and abetted the physician's practices. Not doing a history or a physical—but billing for them and other services unrendered—is felonious fraud and abuse, plain and simple.

Entering wrong diagnoses as a consequence of not following usual and customary medical practices and then ordering inappropriate medications with "black box" warnings (i.e., medications that could cause catastrophic survival outcomes) constitutes additional prosecutorial malpractice. I'll list and discuss the people to whom I sent letters after I describe her second rehab facility.

I had gotten the names of two follow-up rehab facilities. My son-in-law's mother had had the misfortune of using the first. We eliminated that one right off the bat. We notified the second one, and a case interviewer from the rehab facility reviewed the records and interviewed my wife. Joan was accepted and transported. Again, I was assigned a physician without consultation or a discussion of any kind. I only met that physician once. He did not seek me out. I asked one of the nurses when he would be making his appearance. "He usually makes his rounds about nine a.m.," the nurse responded.

I got there at eight. I asked the receptionist, who was located directly at the front entrance, to find me when he arrived. At approximately twelve thirty, I spotted a man standing at the nurse's station in a short-sleeved sport shirt and slacks. He was just making small talk with two techs. I asked his name and verified that he was my wife's assigned physician. No one had notified me of his arrival or notified him that I wanted to see him. I assumed he knew that my wife was a new patient and that he knew his responsibilities for completing and charting the medical intake requirements. This was the last time I would assume anything.

I introduced myself and explained my wife's cognitive problems; I listed her medications for him. He took no notes and did not suggest that we see my wife in her room. He seemed to have some sort of attention deficit disorder. He did not look at me when I spoke. Instead his eyes wandered around the central nurse's station. When I asked for his card, he snapped back into my presence. He could not find one in his pockets or wallet, but he did find one of his fliers in a promotional rack on the wall. "Just call the number on the brochure, twenty-four seven," he said with a broad smile.

I never saw him again. When I tried to contact him, I got an answering service or his office manager. No one ever answered my messages. I complained to the head nurse that my wife did not have chronic obstructive lung disease, nor did she have GERD (gastrointestinal reflux disease); medications prescribed for those conditions were unnecessary, I told her, and contraindicated with her other medications. I told her that I had sent several messages to the assigned physician to correct this problem. She promised to follow up. The chart never changed.

The obvious question you might ask: Why was I allowing this to continue? The answer: the primary reason for her being there was rehabilitation for her repaired right wrist and right hip. That one hour, twice a day, seven days a week, was good...except for New Year's Day. I was surprised to see that they provided physical therapy that day. The Medicare-allowed payment was too good to pass up. But on that morning a new person, in her thirties, showed up. Since she was new, I explained to her that Joan had cognitive problems so that she could take Joan's responses accordingly. The therapist cheerfully looked at me and asked, "On which side did she have her stroke?"

"She did *not* have a stroke," I responded. "She broke her right wrist and right hip.

This obviously didn't faze the therapist.

She pulled the bed covers back with a flourish and continued with a broad smile: "Well, we can take care of that, too."

She either was still celebrating New Year's Eve and/or was smoking her breakfast. I closely monitored Joan's therapy that day and reported it the next day to the head physical therapist.

"That was a contract worker we hired for the day. Thanks for telling us."

At the end of that week (early Friday morning), two nurses and an administrative person confronted me in the hall outside Joan's room. "Joan has been very disruptive," the administrative person announced. "You'll have to hire a sitter."

"What are you talking about; what's a 'sitter'?" I asked.

I was handed three brochures. "It's for your wife's safety. You need someone to watch her twenty-four seven. Medicare does not cover that. She has been getting up and wandering around."

"Why haven't you told me before this, and why haven't I been included in your staff meetings? I'm not only her husband with power of attorney; I'm also a licensed physician."

The broken-record-response continued: "It's for your wife's safety."

Joan's phantom physician, or his representative, had ordered Seroquel (generic name, quetiapine) to try to promote nighttime sedation. The package insert carries a black box warning: "Antipsychotic drugs are associated with an increased risk of death. Quetiapine is not approved for elderly patients with dementia-related psychosis." In addition, psychiatrists informed me that quetiapine is known to have a "paradoxical" dose-related prescribing effect. In other words, if the common starting dose is 25 mg and the patient doesn't show the desired nighttime sedation effect (he or she may even get more agitated), you don't increase the dose, you decrease it by half. When they first put Joan on this medication early after her admission to the facility, I did register my opposition to the head nurse; I also left several messages to that effect with the assigned physician. No one changed the orders.

Back to our conversation. "What if I don't hire a sitter?" I asked.

"Then we'll discharge her; it's for her own safety."

"I'm not sure what you mean by 'discharge' her. Are you going to put her out on the street, or what? Should I call the media now? And when am I supposed to hire a sitter?"

"You have to do it this morning. It's for your wife's safety."

"Which one of these three brochures should I call?"

"We can't tell you that by law. We can only tell you what's available."

One of the nurses made a gesture that she concealed from the others. She raised her index finger to indicate the first brochure out of the three I was holding in my hand. That happened to be the least expensive option: fifteen dollars an hour instead of twenty-five an hour. You do the math: it's a lot of money. What do people do if they don't have the money?

I called the number on the brochure of the advertised family-owned service with a long history of high-quality care, as they put it. The sitter was at the facility in less than an hour. She wanted $5,000 up front.

"I can't cover that on my credit card or my checking account," I lied.

"Can you cover $1,800?"

I played the game and thought for a moment. "Yes," I responded. I roughly calculated that this figure would cover a week or more. She confirmed verbally that I would get a refund for any unused money. I never got a ninety-two dollar owed refund despite several unanswered phone calls and a registered letter. When I made the contract with the sitter service I knew I would be taking Joan out of the rehab facility as soon as I could find a group home or memory care facility. As a matter of record I did eliminate the Seroquel, and Joan did not wander at night. It took a long time and lots of paperwork, but as far as I know, Medicare did not pay the $25,000 to $30,000 for her five-week stay. It wasn't because of my allegations, per se; it was on a technicality. The facility did not have the documentation that Medicare asked for.

Again, I had several locator services to choose from: clearly, this was another thriving business sector. One of the physical therapists swore me to secrecy when he recommended one particular person. My daughter accompanied me, and we decided on the first group home we inspected. It was $5,500 a month, with an extra month's partially refundable deposit. Half would go to the nonrefundable buy-in (called a "community fee"), while the other half would be refundable when Joan left the facility. There were other out-of-pocket expenses, including medications, disposable pull-ups, personal hygiene items, and foot care. Medicare did allow for physical therapy, cognitive work (psychology), and a mandatory monthly physician visit as long as the justification papers were properly filled out. Once we made the group home selection and the manager of the home had interviewed and accepted Joan, I informed the rehab facility that Joan would be discharged the next morning. I told them that I wanted a complete copy of her record.

"We can't do that," I was told. "It takes time to get the orders from the attending physician."

"That's your problem," I responded.

Miraculously, I had a copy of her record and a discharge signature (not the assigned physician's signature) the next morning. The transfer was made.

The manager at the ten-person group home was very experienced and genuinely interested in her work. We developed a very close working relationship after our initial meeting, at which I clearly stated my goals for Joan. The following were important to me:

1. food and fluid intake;
2. daily hygiene;
3. accurate medications; and
4. good communication with myself and family members.

I made it clear that I would not hold the facility responsible for any falls. After all, I had been standing right next to her when she fell and broke her wrist and hip. I knew the challenges and limitations the care home faced and I knew that at some point she would require the next level of care. The communication was excellent, and the manager ensured that any medical concerns I had were quickly known to the physician of record. The staff members were very caring, and it truly felt like *home.* The day did come (the beginning of the seventh month) when we both realized that Joan needed a higher level of care. She was transferred to a memory care facility in Scottsdale. The facility happened to have the same head nurse and physician as the previous care home, which meant that she would have good continuity of medical care. Joan adjusted very well and appeared to like the larger number of patients at the new facility.

After I discharged Joan from the second rehab facility, I had to make a decision relative to reporting fraud and abuse. I was not looking to make money or to get reimbursement of any kind. The question was: Do I do the right thing and report deliberate, calculated fraud and abuse, or do I look the other way? Medicare and my secondary insurance, United Health, would take care of the bills. Joan was still alive, so I could not claim wrongful death. I could include pain and suffering, however, along with the fraud and abuse.

I called a legal office in Phoenix that advertised heavily for clients. I was pleasantly surprised by the considerate reception and timely access I was granted to discussing my situation with a real attorney. In Nevada I had very, very rarely gotten past the front desk to speak with an attorney. The lawyer in Arizona listened carefully and asked me several questions. I knew what the answer would be, and he did not disappoint me: "We cannot take the case, even though it has merit and we would probably win in court. The reality is that winning would not even come close to paying for our time and effort. You can take it to civil court, but without damages, in our opinion, you would be wasting a lot of time and money."

"I thank you for your time and candor," I responded. "I will report it to Medicare, my secondary insurance carrier, and the appropriate licensing boards in Arizona for the two physicians and the two rehabilitation facilities."

The investigations are in progress. The appearance of billing copies from the physicians and rehab facilities stopped shortly after my written complaints. The Arizona Board of Medical Examiners (MD licensing) responded with case numbers. Medicare immediately referred me to its hired contractor, Livanta. United Health thanked me for reporting. I also called the *Arizona Republic*, a leading newspaper in southern Arizona. I spoke to a reporter who had written articles on the Veteran Hospital scandal that was making national news at the time and that had led to the resignation of retired General Shinseki, head of the Department of Veteran Affairs. "I'm very busy with the Phoenix VA story," the reporter told me, "but here's the name and phone number of another reporter you can contact."

I called that reporter, told him my story, and faxed him copies of most of what he requested. He never got back to me as promised, nor would he respond to follow-up phone calls and e-mails.

There used to be a song called "Where Have All the Flowers Gone?" I think they should write another song: "Where Has Journalistic Professionalism and Common Courtesy Gone?"

The final word with all my written complaints was that everyone was declared free of wrongdoing except for the second rehab facility. As stated, Medicare refused to pay (as far as I can ascertain) somewhere between $25 and $30,000 for Joan's five-week stay. Medicare did that solely on technical grounds (and without rendering an opinion on quality of care) and asked the facility for certain documentation—which the facility does not appear to have been able to produce.

Would I do all the work of reporting if I had known the obvious lack of due diligence on the part of the Arizona regulatory bodies? Definitely *yes*! We have a duty to report, even if the odds for an appropriate investigation are slim to none.

CHAPTER **IV**

PERCEPTIONS AND BEHAVIOR—EACH CASE UNTO ITSELF

Are we better off today than post-World War II? Many families do not live within yesteryear's easy proximity of one another. The older folks live where the children grew up, while the children have scattered, depending on educational and job opportunities. Everything moves at a faster pace, which leaves less time for family socialization and the exchange of ideas and perhaps helpful advice for those inevitable life-altering decisions that must eventually be made—let alone the physical presence to lend a hand during unexpected emergencies.

We've accumulated technology galore in an effort to become more efficient, make more money, and have greater discretionary wealth and time to enjoy it. Have we succeeded? We live longer, but have we adequately planned to take care of the unintended consequences, such as providing caregiving at all age levels? Have we lost some of our *soul* by listening to one another less?

The business world in the United States emphasizes fee for service, free trade, talks about work ethics, and the pursuit of the American Dream. At least those are some of the sound bites. Then there are those endeavors like religion, health care, and teaching, where standards are more like following the golden rule, turning the other cheek, and giving for the general good. At least those phrases have not been forgotten. A case could be made, however, that the oft-stated constitutional right to life, liberty, and the pursuit of happiness has become overshadowed by too great a pursuit of money and possessions. The obsessive pursuit of wealth changes how we think, act, and relate. Unfortunately, health care is no exception. Good intentions for safe and healthy work and living spaces have led to increased rules and regulations, but what can be said of the application and oversight? The same applies for improving social services for those at the bottom of our socioeconomic pyramid. The opening question to this chapter remains: Overall, have we made things better?

Below are a few case examples of current health-care practices and omissions that could use some corrective attention. This is obviously the tip of the iceberg. Anticipatory guidance (i.e., planning ahead) is far better than waiting for emergency catchup. Expect setbacks, disappointments, and dead ends, but without continuously trying to make things better, we guarantee failure—and failure is never an option.

Case One: Beware of Casual Advice

There was a time when writing a book, giving a talk, or engaging in one-on-one interaction with a caregiver/advocate carried little to no legal overtones. Now, more often than not, authors and speakers include disclaimers such as "The material offered here does not constitute actual or implied responsibility for actions and outcomes, or lack thereof." Defensive medical practices have become the norm. Similarly, the public at large has adopted similar disclaimers, including being politically correct and/or not rocking the boat.

My wife, as noted earlier, was an avid bridge player. She met a very friendly woman in the course of her card-playing days who had moved from Reno to Las Vegas. Her husband was a tennis player. I got to know him on the courts as we played, and we discussed some of our common interests. One day they invited us as their guests to a show at the Golden Nugget Hotel on Fremont Street in downtown Las Vegas. Their son was a talented music arranger and piano player for a very popular show. We had a nice evening and reciprocated by paying for dinner after the show. During dinner, the wife pointed to a bump on her forehead. "Should I do anything about this?" she asked.

Like most doctors, I don't enjoy rendering medical opinions outside of a professional setting. Not wishing to be insensitive, I asked her a few questions about the lump's history before giving her a list of possibilities. I ended with my standard caveat: "You can't be sure of what it is unless it is biopsied, and you definitely need to have that done without delay. I can give you the names of one or two physicians that I would see if I were in your shoes."

Nothing was written down, since I'm not in the habit of carrying records to dinner. She thanked me and did not pursue my referral offer. Six to eight weeks later I met her husband on the tennis courts. I asked how he, his wife, and their musical son were doing. He responded in an angry tone. "My wife has a serious lymphoma type of cancer. You told her not to worry about it when we had dinner that night."

"Whoa!" I interrupted. "I never said that. I said that it could be anything from a fatty tumor to something more serious; I specifically advised her to have it biopsied without delay. I also offered to give her the names of physicians I myself would go to. I'm sorry to hear about her diagnosis."

We remain tennis friends, but I don't think he ever altered his recall of what in his mind I had allegedly said to his wife that night. It was necessary that I reconsider my practice of freely responding to requests for medical opinions and/or referrals.

Case Two: Documentation—A Corollary to Case One

Our retirement community has several recreation centers. I ride my bike to the one closest to our rental home. A couple in their late seventies regularly work out in that facility. The husband, who is clearly the dominant partner in that relationship, seems to have selective hearing in that he appears to automatically reject anything that challenges his perceptions. As a consequence, whenever we see each other in the locker room we greet each other but discuss nothing. If I see his wife in the lobby, I say hello and she responds with averted eye contact and a whispered *hello*. On one occasion, as the husband was about to leave the locker room, he abruptly stopped and asked: "Can you recommend a neurologist for my wife? She has a balance problem."

I should have asked a few questions, such as how long has she had the balance problem? Was it sudden or gradual onset? Is she being seen for any other medical problems? I did not want to appear as if I were soliciting as a consultant, however, so I said: "Write down your e-mail address, and I'll send you one or two names with their contact information." I did that when I returned home, and he thanked me by return e-mail.

One or two days later our paths crossed once more in the locker room, and he again thanked me. He casually added: "It may be a while before I call the neurologist. She just finished up with Dr. Jameson [not his true name]. She likes him."

Whoa, I thought to myself; he is a surgeon. Aloud I said, "Yeah, he is a nice guy and a very good surgeon. What was that all about?"

"He took out a large melanoma." He pointed to his lower left abdomen, just above his groin.

"I'm sure he told you to follow up with a cancer specialist," I said.

"Yes, he mentioned something about a skin and cancer group, but for now she has no sign of the melanoma."

It was obvious that he had selectively heard what he wanted to hear from Dr. Jameson. I know Dr. Jameson as a very well-read meticulous surgeon, and I'm sure he told this man that his wife needed an immediate follow-up for the latest immunotherapy that former president Jimmy Carter was receiving for his wide-spread melanoma at the time, including brain metastasis.

I explained: "You must have been preoccupied with your wife's diagnosis so that you didn't get the full picture from Dr. Jameson. I know the doc, and he always takes time to explain your options. Melanoma is notorious for spreading, and even though he removed a large mass for control of local problems, I guarantee that your wife still has melanoma in her body. The only chance of remission is immunotherapy. Time is critical. You have to see a tumor specialist, not a neurologist—an oncologist."

I gave him the name of an oncology group, mentioned Jimmy Carter, and stressed the importance of immediate consultation with the oncology group. I went home and repeated all of the information via e-mail, including the fact that he should request immunotherapy and that he should use my name as a referent if he wished. I also explained why I was taking the time to send the e-mail: "I know you are under a lot of stress from coping with your wife's medical problem. It's hard enough remembering our everyday chores let alone new challenges. I'm writing this down as a permanent record so that you have exactly what Dr. Jameson and I recommend. I stress the importance of doing this without delay. I'd appreciate your letting me know if you encounter any problems with the oncology group. I can't be involved as part of your wife's medical team, but I can help you find the people who are best qualified to treat her."

The take-home message of this is that if you are a caregiver or advocate or are in any way responsible for another person's activities of daily living, make sure that you try to organize, document, and be proactive everything you can. It does require time and perseverance, but it's crucial that you do this.

Case Three: Empathy and Sensitivity

Shortly after my wife's transfer to a higher level of memory care, I found myself adjusting to the modern version of old Hollywood depictions of caring for cognitively impaired patients. In those days they were called mentally ill, or "just plain crazy." The very violent were separated from the rest in padded cells (in locked isolation), while the rest were managed with as-needed sedatives: usually barbiturates. That was the norm during my medical internship at a New York county hospital in 1957. Today we have better medications but also more undesirable side effects and astronomic expenses. The patient population is very ethnically diverse, as is the staff. We have dedicated people with huge variations in abilities and training. The staff come from Central and South America, West Africa, Asia, and Europe. The United States has been called the melting pot of the world. Cognitively impaired care facilities are the extension of that pot, and in many respects I consider these facilities to be a fourth-world type of country-within-a-country. I had arrived early, intending to help the staff serve breakfast. I greeted my wife with a hug and a kiss. She smiled and said: "I am going to take a nap."

"No," I replied. "They are getting breakfast ready. Do you want to sit at the same table as yesterday?"

She smiled and replied in the affirmative, but she was heading back to her room.

"Breakfast is over there," I said.

Her confused stare disappeared as instantaneously as it had appeared. She greeted everyone at the breakfast table. Joan ate with gusto and chatted aimlessly with her tablemates. I asked if she would like to take a walk around her secured wing of the facility.

"After I take a nap," she replied.

I walked her to her room, got her comfortable, gave her a kiss, and told her that I'd be back in the evening. I thanked the staff, took a deep breath, and headed out through the locked doors. There was a time when I might have dwelled on Joan's thoughts, actions, and confusions. Now I gratefully accept a problem-free visit with *some sadness, some serenity, and lots of acceptance.*

A newcomer gentleman was in my path to the car. He was staring into the clear morning sky as he smoked a cigarette. His whole being exuded painful loneliness.

"Another beautiful morning in the Southwest," I said.

"Yes," he replied with a sigh, a smoky exhalation, and a Hispanic accent.

I was in no rush so I asked where he was from.

"Argentina," he told me.

I told him I was a physician and that my wife was a patient in the memory care facility. He told me his wife had been newly admitted. We compared notes, and it was obvious that I was relatively better off of the two of us.

He was a retired engineer who had come to Arizona with his wife to be near their only son and his family. The adjustment to their new environment had been going well for about three years when his wife began to exhibit signs of dementia. The husband took over the chores of shopping, laundry, preparing meals, and monitoring her dressing and hygiene. The doctors had told him that his wife's problems were most likely due to circulatory complications from diabetes, hypertension, and bad cholesterol. To add to his situation, the son and his family had recently had a job transfer to California. Now he was on his own; he had no insurance to cover the tremendous medical and custodial costs involved. He was in the country on a visa and had submitted an application for citizenship. I gave him my card and assured him that I was not looking for clients. I volunteered a few ideas he might want to explore and told him to call me with any questions that I might be able to answer. I knew there wasn't much I could really do, but the chance for him to talk to someone might have provided him with a ray of hope.

If you're the caregiver, don't be shy about engaging strangers for help and for venting. If you're a stranger, don't be shy about offering a compassionate ear.

Case Four: The Accountant

For a short period of time I took my wife to a Las Vegas day-care center. The place was located in the poorer section of town in an old building with a predominance of welfare (Medicaid) patients. I was particularly interested in their Friday morning program, in which they selected no more than twelve mixed-gender people with mild to moderate cognitive impairment and removed them to a separate room. The idea was to engage the group in discussions, arts and crafts, and whatever else the specially trained two-person staff could create for thought and interactive stimulation. The rest of the clientele were in the main room, where most stared at a large TV set, stared at one another, or stared into space. Some had closed their eyes and retreated into whatever world remained for them. A few aimlessly wandered around in various states of restlessness, danced by themselves to imaginary music, or delivered abstract oratory to a nonexistent audience. In plain words, it was a pathetic zoo for human warehousing. If you weren't on welfare, or possibly some type of insurance, the fee was eighty dollars per day, from eight in the morning to five in the afternoon. They provided breakfast and lunch with afternoon snacks.

Joan enjoyed the small group but did not want to stay very long after lunch in the large main "zoo" area. The facility had musical entertainers in the afternoon, but after fifteen minutes she was ready to return home. She never said anything about the mixed group, but she made it clear that she wanted me there no later than 1:00 p.m. so that she could leave.

The same administrative group ran a sister operation in nearby Henderson on Wednesdays, and, although it meant a forty-mile round-trip, I decided to give it a try. The building and facilities were essentially new, and the clientele was decidedly middle to upper class. Joan liked that facility better but soon tired of that, too. I paid cash for each session.

I had noticed a man dropping his wife off at the downtown Friday sessions, and she, too, was anxious to leave right after lunch. In fact, she was always sitting near the door when I came to get Joan and she would ask me for a ride, even though she didn't know me or where I was going. Her husband lived in the same retirement community as me; he worked out daily in our recreation center. He asked about my wife, and we had discussions about our needs, goals, and challenges. He was particularly stressed with his wife's progressive incontinence. I voiced my decision that if Joan developed that problem, she would be going into some level of a care facility. I could not handle that challenge, even with home-help visits. I pointed out that his current state of stress was not helping him or his wife; he agreed that he had been short-tempered with everything she did or did not do. Eventually he told me that he had come to terms with his guilt feelings about putting his wife into a care facility. I had canvassed a lot of facilities in the Las Vegas area in anticipation of needing one for Joan. When he mentioned which facility he had chosen, I was surprised, since I thought it was poorly run with minimally trained personnel. He visited daily even though she had ceased to recognize him or her surroundings. She passed away within two months. I tried to mitigate his obvious guilt about his decisions for terminal care.

"I hope you realize, you had no choice but to put her in a care facility. You took care of her at home for as long you could and then some. She was obviously running out of time. Yes, some professionals will say that people seem to 'decompensate' faster when they are institutionalized. I say that that's irrelevant when the caregiver is faced with impossible challenges at home. It's no different than caring for any person with a terminal disease: you make the person as comfortable as possible and have her experience end of life with dignity. When the time comes and she passes on, don't rush the readjustments. Covet the good memories of a life well spent and move on to gather more good experiences."

The husband might have taken my advice. He disappeared from his daily workout at the recreation center. Someone told me he had met a girlfriend and had moved closer to one of his children.

Case Five: Just the Two of Them

Change is frequently difficult, especially as we get older and have adapted to conditions we've accepted as comfortable and workable. As youngsters, we don't think about life-changing challenges. While we can't plan for every adverse possibility, realistic anticipatory planning is available and doable. Mary and John (real people, but not their real names) are more common than we'd like to admit. They never had children, and the few relatives they did have were not close. Now, with both of them at age ninety, there are no relatives: just the two of them living by themselves in a retirement community. They never went out for meals and rarely went to social events. John had worked as a supervisor in the oil industry, and Mary took care of the house. The pension and Medicare covered their simple lifestyle.

Mary, at just under five feet and maybe seventy-five pounds with wet clothes, has found it increasingly difficult to help John bathe, dress, and shop. They eat prefrozen meals. John's pacemaker corrected his dizzy spells but made it clear that his circulation was slowly failing along with his memory, concentration, verbal communication, and thought processes. Her family physician had periodically mentioned the need for a trust, will, and power of attorney, and thought about selling the house and going into assisted living. He also told her she should not be driving, get help to take care of John, clean the house, and talk to a lawyer and/or estate planner about the future.

You know the rest: family physicians are not really family physicians anymore. They are very busy gatekeepers who may or may not give appropriate and timely advice to patients, who are prone to put off following the advice. Patients all too often don't know where to start or whom they can trust. Luckily, her family doctor had had to make a house call for John (also a rare happening in city-type living), and when he saw how much help Mary needed (but was too proud to ask for), he made it a point to have qualified professionals come to the house to discuss and plan for medical, legal, and economic needs. It's easy to say the words but very difficult to make it happen. Consider the following two headlines: "Privacy's Double-Edged Sword: Families Are Cut Out" and "Law Leaves Loved Ones of Mentally Ill Patients on the Sidelines— Sometimes With Tragic Results."

If you are a caregiver/advocate, pay close attention to timely planning, be relentless in pursuit of honest and qualified professionals, and always report any wrongdoing. If you're a neighbor and/or real friend, become the *right stuff and go out of your way to actually help*. Your turn may come and you would want no less.

Chapter V

IS IT JUST SOMETHING AGE APPROPRIATE?

"The Man in the Glass"
Peter Dale Wimbrow Sr.

When you get what you want in your struggle for self
And the world makes you king for a day
Just go to the mirror and look at yourself
And see what that man has to say.

For it isn't your father, or mother, or wife
Whose judgment upon you must pass
The fellow whose verdict counts most in your life
Is the one staring back from the glass.

He's the fellow to please—never mind all the rest
For he's with you, clear to the end
And you've passed your most difficult, dangerous test
If the man in the glass is your friend.

You may fool the whole world down the pathway of years
And get pats on the back as you pass
But your final reward will be heartache and tears
If you've cheated the man in the glass.

This poem was first published in 1934 and is still very popular today. Thank you very much to the family of Dale Wimbrow for allowing us to publish it and to my daughter, Kay Segal, for recommending it.

I debated using real names and places in this book but finally opted to let it all hang out. There is no intent to embarrass or incite lawsuits. I recognize and applaud the good intentions of those who are genuinely trying to improve the world. It is called *tikkum olam* in Hebrew: repairing the world. I hope the following true narrative will be taken as something that constructively shines a light on what needs to be corrected in the system. We can and must do better, because what we are doing is both economically unsustainable and medically counterproductive for patient well-being.

I had lunch with an eighty-year-old friend of mine who looks like a twin of actors Yul Brynner or Telly Savalas (of *Kojak* fame), both of whom are totally and smoothly bald. We have a lot in common. He grew up in New York, has the same religious back ground as me, and was educated as a chemical engineer but became an accountant, and lawyer. He finally became a judge in California. Upon retirement he purchased a second home in an eight-thousand-home retirement community in Las Vegas's Sun City Summerlin. We enjoy discussing each other's philosophies, areas of expertise, and the news *de jour*. Occasionally we discussed medications.

At one particular lunch I brought along the package insert of an antipsychotic medication prescribed for my wife by other physicians. The entire insert, unfolded, could easily fit into three to four pages of a major newspaper, in small print no less. I pointed to the black box warning, which underlined in bold black letters that it could cause serious side effects, including death, especially in patients like my wife who had a history of bipolarism. Among the long list of side effects, I highlighted *hypotension* (a drop in blood pressure), which could cause unconsciousness and falls. Injuries from falls in the elderly, especially women, are among the leading causes of disability and death. Indeed, my wife was falling quite often, with consequent serious injuries.

"Well," my lunch companion said. "Everything is a trade-off: risk versus benefit."

I agreed and responded: "But in this case my professional opinion was based on knowing my wife's medical history better than anyone else and in addition devoting time to carefully reading the package inserts of all medications. I had only one patient and plenty of time to direct my focus. The medication in question was very likely the cause of her passing out when she stood up. We had better alternatives to treat her 'agitated depression' characterized by poor sleep patterns and a tendency to wander the locked premises."

My friend looked puzzled. "Joan is lucky. You are a very qualified physician and you have power of attorney. You can discuss it with Joan's professional team. If they don't agree with your analysis and wishes, you can still act on your own."

"Ah, don't I wish."

Now the door was open for me to vent, and I appreciated his interest and intellect. "The entire system is broke, *kaput*! All over the country, bean counters, nonphysicians, and gamers with conflicts of interest have taken control of health care. Here is an example of a typical office visit. I walk into a doctor's office with Joan, and the doctor opens his laptop and starts entering data. He has to follow the protocol or he won't get paid. He pays little attention to the patient (Joan) or the caregiver (me). Since Joan can't reliably answer questions, her team (physicians, nursing personnel, and technicians) should be speaking and listening to me. When all is said and done I get a printed summary of what allegedly transpired at that visit. It is given to me by a clerk at the exit desk. Invariably, parts of that summary are totally incorrect, because the physician or his or her proxy (nurse practitioner or physician assistant) wasn't talking to me while making eye contact, let alone brain contact. To make matters worse, by the time I get the summary at the front desk, the physician has disappeared to whatever is next on his or her schedule. It is impossible for me—even though I am a licensed medical professional—to contact the physician directly and discuss the patient, my wife. There is no e-mail address or dedicated phone line for medical colleagues. I have to leave my message with an office manager, program coordinator, or maybe the front-desk clerk. Most of the time there is no feedback. I have to wait for the next appointment and hope that nothing crucial happens in the interim. If something crucial *does* happen, I get the familiar recording:'If this is an emergency, hang up and call 911.' For sure, there are exceptions, but my experience with a few of the big-name centers indicates trends toward exclusion of the primary-care physician from participating in his patient's care, and it hasn't mattered that I am the patient's physician-husband who has power of attorney. I swear I'm not exaggerating! If I'm having these problems, how do nonprofessional caregivers cope?"

I went on to cite, as examples, departments in the University of Nevada School of Medicine (UNSOM) and the Cleveland Clinic's Lou Ruvo Center for Brain Health. My friend was well aware of Joan's cognitive medical history, so I proceeded to tell him about my experiences with Joan at the Brain Center. I acknowledged that the philanthropist Larry Ruvo, following his father's (Lou Ruvo's) battle with Alzheimer's, had been motivated to establish a center in Las Vegas to pursue research and clinical applications in degenerative diseases of the brain. He successfully accomplished that monumental task and he deserves the greatest recognition for doing so. In my opinion, however, the professionals who operate the system are missing the mark, especially when it comes to including and encouraging local professional participation, as I stated above related to local physicians' lack of access to staff physicians. Several other critical areas deserve scrutiny, and Mr. Ruvo can't be expected to recognize those areas on his own. Unfortunately, the medical experts in his inner circle don't appear to be particularly anxious about burdening him with what they appear to consider their exclusive professional domain. I went on to describe my wife's visits to the Brain Center. My friend continued to pay very close attention.

"In 2009," I told him, "I got a copy of *New Thinking* in the mail—the quarterly magazine the Brain Center puts out. I read about their clinical trials. I thought that maybe Joan could be enrolled in a research protocol for her benefit and/or for scientific advancement. I made several phone calls to the center, received papers to fill out, and was finally told that she did not qualify for any of the cognitive protocols, since she had the additional diagnosis of bipolar disease. I was puzzled by the lack of interest in that particular condition, since it relates to the later onset of cognitive impairment. When I ask neurologists at the Brain Center and elsewhere about that lack of interest, I get responses along the lines of: 'Yeah, it appears that maybe there is a greater incidence of cognitive impairment in people with bipolar disease.'"

But no one gives me definitive studies, past or present, and I haven't been able to find relative studies through the Internet. The reason, in my opinion, is that there isn't enough money in it to motivate pharmaceutical companies to fund research, and not enough people are interested to ask for government funding from the NIH.

I continued to explain my story to my lawyer friend: "I had ongoing discussions with my psychiatrist son about his mother's cognitive medical care, since he had made the original diagnosis. I had gotten a PET-CT scan of the brain, which showed no definitive markers for any type of dementia. Her diagnosis was: mild to moderate cognitive impairment. It had a specific medical billing code number that meant that they did not know the cause (etiology). I was in the sixth or seventh year of her care in our home setting at this point. I decided that maybe I should see a neurologist at the Brain Center just to make sure we weren't missing anything. I made an appointment to see a neurologist whom I casually knew from his time at the teaching hospital in southern Nevada. He asked me questions and entered my answers into his laptop. He then reviewed the medical realities of what I already knew and told me: 'I'd like to get an MRI, sleep study test, psychology evaluation, and baseline laboratory tests.'

"At this I sighed and puckered my lips in momentary thought. 'We just had the PET-CT scan of the brain,' I told him, 'and it showed nothing of value. You have the report and images, along with the laboratory tests. She is already on the Aricept and Namenda that our son had put her on. Incidentally, based on my review of the data, I don't think those medications have any real value. Why not leave all the testing out? We can come back in six months for a clinical follow-up.'"

"The neurologist responded. 'We like to get our baselines, so to speak.'"

I continued with my story. "I reluctantly allowed him to order approximately $15,000 worth of billable studies. Medicare and my secondary insurance paid the reduced contract allowances, but nothing of value was obtained from the studies. I did not return. One of the main reasons I did not return was that the neurologist kept pushing for a diagnosis of Alzheimer's, and I was convinced that she did hot have Alzheimer's; even if I had gone along with his diagnosis of Alzheimer's, it would not have provided any new treatment options. Another annoying result of that one patient visit for my wife was our addition to the endless marketing literature from Cleveland Clinic in Ohio."

I continued. "About three years later [in 2012] I received my periodic copy of *New Thinking* from the Brain Center, which included an article that heralded the addition of a new physician who would be specializing in fronto-temporal dementia, among other things. Since my working diagnosis for Joan was that type of dementia, I decided to give it another try. After about $50,000 more of billable services and procedures, with unnecessary demands in time and personal expense and nothing to gain from it, I terminated the visits."

My lunch companion interrupted: "What was the name of the second doctor you saw?"

I repeated the name and asked, "Have you see him?"

"Yes, Linda [his wife] suggested that I get checked for Alzheimer's, because she noticed I was having a few senior moments. What you're telling me about Joan's experience is very disturbing to me."

"Why?" I asked.

"Well, the doctor took the history and put it all into his laptop. He ordered the brain imaging tests [MRI and PET-CT scans], the sleep study, and the three-hour psychological evaluation, and they took buckets of blood for lab tests. I have never seen so many vials of blood taken from me at one time. It sounds like some type of cookbook routine, and I'm not sure of the end-game value. It won't cost me out-of-pocket but it will take time and cause inconvenience, and to what end?"

"OK, let me summarize," I replied. "I happened to notice that you'd been a little slower in processing a few thoughts and recalling items when we'd met during the last year or two. I wasn't sure whether it might be due to decreased hearing or just a normal age-related decrease in response time: our so-called senior moments. I didn't say anything, because it was obvious that you were still carrying on with all your activities of daily living, which is actually a very active routine for being eighty. I can't fault you or your wife for wondering if you are headed for a miserable end-of-life scenario. You responded to the media hype and direct-marketing strategists, just like they wanted you to. But consider these facts." I proceeded to tell him the following list.

1. All of these tests most likely will not reveal a definitive diagnosis.
2. If they do come up with a diagnosis of Alzheimer's or some other dementia, what can they offer the patient?
3. Only two medications are available: Namenda tablets and Aricept tablets (or the patch version from another company). The drug companies admit that neither one will stop the disease, but they say "it may slow the progression." I told my friend that my professional conclusion did not support either drug's use in any type of dementia. In addition, some physicians have cautioned against a rapid decline in some patients when Namenda or Aricept is discontinued. This suggests the possibility that either of the drugs, or when given in combination, may cause some sort of addiction or dependence. I told my friend to read the side effects warning and then decide if he would take either one in light of a risk/benefit consideration.
4. I told him that they may be able to enter him into a research protocol, which would be a noble consideration.
5. I told him that they can give him all kinds of mumbo jumbo about eating healthy, exercising regularly, taking

the "amazing protein Prevagen" (as advertised on television) extracted from jellyfish and shown by scientists (none identified) to improve memory, loading up on antioxidants, having more sex, drinking more red wine, doing yoga and meditation, enrolling in "brain exercise" courses, taking a cruise, or developing a hobby—you name it. You've heard the expression: "Use it or lose it." We all know that the driving factor for all of this is money in somebody's pocket. What people may not know, I told my friend, is that food additives, supplements, and devices like magnets and copper bracelets do not come under the regulation of the FDA. The additive and supplement advertising is very cleverly worded to minimize or totally escape legal accountability.

6. Finally, I told my friend, there is a gray area of ethical, moral, and legal accountability in all this. One can argue that when he went to the brain center to try to find out if his senior moments were just age-appropriate happenings that were of no consequence or perhaps something worse, was his physician justified in running a series of expensive and time-consuming procedures in order to come to the best possible conclusion and offer the best advice? Very creditable physicians have stated that 85–90 percent of diagnoses can be made accurately with a good history and physical examination. As I told my friend, our psychiatrist son concluded on a diagnosis of very early dementia with a simple fifteen-minute word test (the aforementioned Mini-Cog) in his office. Nothing else was needed. Furthermore, Medicare and other insurance money is intended for clinical applications, which means diagnoses and treatments and not research that collects data and hopes that a discovery will miraculously fall into their laps. If they have a credible research idea in mind, then they should apply for research grant money. In light of what I explained earlier

about the paucity of meaningful treatments for dementias, is the Brain Center (or similar centers in the United States) justified in the willy-nilly collection of very expensive data and possibly writing reports at some point in the future? The report would most likely say something along the lines of: "The findings are very suggestive of this or that and merit further studies." That's a not-too-subtle way of pursuing job security by continuing to syphon money from the clinical application pot to a sham research pot. Research is supposed to be supported by governmental grants, philanthropic grants, or industry-driven grants, and there are specific procedures for applying.

We finished lunch. I asked my friend to go home and look up the two medications I'd mentioned to him on the Internet. I'd call in an hour or so to see what he thought. "Well," I asked him later that day, "did you read the package inserts?"

"I sure did," he replied, "and you are right. The risks far outweigh any benefits. I'm very upset. I really don't think I'll go back."

"Let me ask you a personal question," I said. "If you were paying for the visits and tests out of your pocket, would you even consider going in the first place, even if they billed on actual reduced Medicare-allowed fees?"

"Hell no!"

"Well, my friend, you have to decide for yourself. Don't tell me what you decide; that's your business. We're all targets of media hype, irrational health-care exuberance, and unabashed fraud and abuse."

If I were his family physician (which is what I did for thirteen years) and my friend had come to me and asked me questions about his senior moments, I would have taken a detailed family and personal history followed by a complete physical examination. I would have administered the simple, fifteen-minute Mini-Cog word test. I then would have explained what further testing could offer (in his case, little to nothing), and I would have recommended no further testing at that time. I would obviously comment on any lifestyle changes if he indeed needed that, such as losing weight, not smoking, and engaging in a reasonable amount of exercise at least three times a week for an hour or so. Would that have reassured him, I asked, or would he want "the works," since it wasn't coming directly out of his pocket?

This is a lot of information to think about, and, like many other things, it probably raises more questions than it answers. It essentially points out that health-care providers have their moral, ethical, and professional responsibilities, and so does the consumer-patient. We may try but we cannot deny mortality. We don't have to create drama and turmoil as is commonly done in the entertainment, economic, and spiritual worlds. Let's try to keep it focused on our constitutional precepts of life, liberty, and the pursuit of happiness—and I don't mean the drug-induced variety of happiness.

CHAPTER VI

EMOTIONS, FACTS, AND DENIALS

I listened to Patrick Kennedy, the son of the late senator Edward Kennedy, talk about his book *Shame Can Kill You*, which highlights at least two cardinal principals related to mental health: 1) poor mental health can seriously affect anyone, regardless of educational or socioeconomic status, and 2) little help will be available if we do not recognize and freely discuss the challenges without shame or inhibitions. His soul-bearing book honestly confronts his personal and collective family conundrums in dealing with life. The author talks about illness, drugs, tragedy, and the ever-present code of silent cover-up. Stories about the Kennedy dynasty are both pervasive and timeless. Let's bring it home to long-standing perceived stigmas of mental illness and the paranoia about keeping it secret.

I joined a group of caregivers that met once a week for about two hours. They shared their thoughts, problems, and good and bad experiences. The moderator was a credentialed social worker who supplied reading materials and kept the discussions moving as best she could. I attended more out of curiosity than personal needs. The attendees represented the entire range of older caregivers: spouses, children, appointed advocates, and longtime friends.

One woman who was in obvious distress was trying to cope with her husband, who was in his late seventies. He had been diagnosed with Alzheimer's approximately seven years earlier. She had been caring for him at home until his behavior toward her became aggressively negative, such as throwing food, verbally and physically challenging her, and wandering around the house at all hours. One weekend, fearing for her safety, she made a call to the neurologist who had been seeing her husband. She got the familiar message in which she was told the office hours and, "If this is an emergency, hang up and call 911." She called 911, and the ambulance arrived.

She provided the physician's name and her husband's diagnosis. The EMTs sedated her husband and transported him to a hospital emergency room where, after an eight-hour wait in the ER, he was admitted to the neurology service with her neurologist as the physician in charge. The neurologist had left orders over the phone but did not show up to see the patient or the patient's wife until after noon the next day. What is your reaction to this true scenario? Should the neurologist, at the very least, have spoken to the wife over the phone?

Back in the 1960s and 70s, primary-care physicians (and the neurologist in this case, who was the patient's primary-care physician in charge of the primary medical condition of Alzheimer's disease) did not sign out to the emergency room. In many rural areas, emergency rooms were covered by primary-care physicians on a rotating call schedule. The usual and customary practice of the primary-care physician was either to be available around the clock, every day of the week, or to provide specific coverage with another physician. With this in mind, you could rightly conclude that medicine has made great advances in technical areas, but not in physician-patient interactions. This is sometimes called the four A's: availability, affordability, affability, and accessibility.

The neurologist in this case met with the wife and assured her that he would be able to control her husband's disruptive behavior with medications, but he further informed her that she would do well to talk to the social-service people about finding an appropriate care facility. He estimated that her husband would be discharged in approximately ten to fourteen days. The pressing question the wife had for the support group was: What she should do about visiting her husband in the hospital? Despite the medications he was now on, every time she visited he would immediately become enraged, hurl verbal abuse at her, and threaten to beat her up if she didn't take him home.

"John was never like that," she told us. "I can't calm him, and the new medications do not seem to be helping. I get very upset and I leave. Then I feel bad about not staying; I wonder if I should give him one more try at home."

The fifteen or so caregivers at the meeting gave her all kinds of advice and anecdotes, but no one provided her with direct answers to her questions about continuing to visit the hospital or taking her husband home. Realistically, how could they? No one really knew the temperament of this woman, her financial situation, what mentoring she had received relative to understanding her husband's disease, or her efforts to plan for legal, financial, and medical decisions. Wouldn't it be nice if her neurologist had taken an hour or so to explain the medical aspects of her husband's disease and then had actually assembled a team to answer her questions and monitor her progress? Some caregivers are blessed with finances, family, and other support groups, as well as a resilient determination to stay engaged. Rarely are caregivers blessed with a well-trained physician who takes the time and makes the effort to coordinate all aspects of medical care.

In all fairness, in today's health-care delivery in the United States, physicians do face huge challenges in managing time, documentation requirements, and various expenses—such as debts from medical school, licensing and malpractice insurance fees, and office expenses—that in some instances run well over 50 percent of the physician's gross income. Some physicians perform better than others, and the person you get during a time of medical need is strictly a matter of luck—and diligently doing your homework.

The next case exemplifies the unrealistic expectations we often have about control, even when we have the funds to cover the care. In this case, the husband-caregiver had total coverage for several months through Medicare and his secondary insurance, but only if his wife was transferred from a hospital setting to a rehabilitation facility. The physicians at the rehabilitation facility controlled the Medicare-covered length of stay by how diligently they followed the Medicare requirements in filling out the periodic progress reports. Needless to say, lots of creative and/or sloppy reporting is done when it comes to insurance requirements.

The husband called me to say, "I saw an article you wrote about health care and caregivers. Can I tell you about my wife and ask your opinion on a few things?"

"Of course," I replied. "Please understand, however, that I'm only rendering an opinion based on my experiences relative to what you tell me; I am not creating a physician-patient relationship. Any opinions I provide are strictly for you to discuss with your primary-care physician. Any actions you take are strictly between you and your health-care providers, and I am not part of that process. That's called 'covering my rear.'"

"Of course," he replied. "I do appreciate your listening and giving me your thoughts. My wife has Alzheimer's (or something like it). I've been taking care of her at home for seven years now. It was a lot of work, since I had to do everything. A few weeks ago she fell and broke her hip. The surgery went well. They even got her out of bed the next day. She had almost two weeks in rehabilitation at the same hospital. They said that she could be transferred to another type of hospital for more rehabilitation, or I could take her home and find help to come to the house through Medicare. Of course, I preferred to take her home. You know, at home I only have her to take care of. All of these nursing homes have lots of patients, and I've heard some bad stories. Well, the home visits are very limited, so I have to plan around what they provide, like going shopping, giving her an extra bath, and of course cleaning her up when she has an accident. It's a lot harder for me now than it was before she broke her hip. She really can't walk without me holding her, so she is in the wheelchair when she is not in bed. I knew I couldn't keep doing this, so I called the social worker at the hospital and explained everything to her. She gave me a few places to check out: you know, like nursing homes. I tell you, I wouldn't put a dog in some of these places. Then I found out that Medicare would not cover any of it, because she is at home and not in a hospital. No one ever told me about that rule. I have an insurance plan that I've been paying for years, and only now do I find out that they only cover about $125 a day for a few months. The real cost for any of these places is closer to $5,000 a month, and that will come out of my pocket."

I listened to his long and familiar story. I assumed that it was helpful for him to have his verbal catharsis. He had no other family, and it sounded like he really had no close friends.

He continued: "I picked a place that was fairly new. I watched one of their movie promotions and listened to a pitch from the head nurse, who was the administrator, too. They showed me a private room and a two-person room, the dining room, the exercise room, and the social room. I transferred my wife without any trouble. I had to pay for the transport. It was like transferring a shell-shocked refugee. She just sat in the wheelchair and said nothing. She didn't even look up at me or at anything else. I tell you. I really felt bad, but I also looked forward to a quiet night for a change. I hired a cleaning crew to show up and clean the house, open the windows, and get rid of that terrible sick smell. I visit my wife every day so that I can help feed her and just be there. I really don't know if she realizes who I am, but I feel like I owe it to her. She has had a few accidents, and I know they can't always clean her up right away, but it is becoming an expected condition every day I show up: she's been lying in her waste for God only knows how long. I asked the attendants to please try to keep a closer watch. I even gave them some cash. They smile and thank me. I finally asked to meet with the nurse-supervisor. You know what she said? She told me, 'We have two hundred beds. We have enough staff to meet state and federal regulations. We are also part of a chain heath-care company that makes us follow a budget. We do the best we can and we know we could do better if we had the money to hire more people. You could hire a full- or part-time sitter/caretaker as a supplement to what we provide.'"

"Well," the husband continued. "I told her that I can't hire a sitter. My budget is already stretched. So my question to you is: Do you have any ideas about what I can do?"

I felt like saying, "Welcome to the real world of acceptance. Accept the fact that you have little to no control at this point in time. Accept the fact that you can't take care of your wife at home. Accept the fact that she will only get worse and not better. Accept the fact that you've done the best you can and maybe even accept the fact that you should look for new relationships and enjoyment without feeling guilty." No, I didn't take that approach with him, but I was ready to discuss those ideas if the conversation went in that direction. I thought that it was most important to give him some of the immediate options that are not always presented (and not always understood when they are presented).

I told him, "I'm not sure you understand how Medicare works (or how people make Medicare work for them). I'm not saying that it is ethical or even legal, nor am I saying that you should take advantage of it. You can think about it and make up your own mind. I also don't know your financial situation and I don't need to know. Medicare will cover rehabilitative extended care if the patient is transferred after three or more days in an acute-care hospital. The physicians involved with rehabilitative care understand the rules of periodic evaluations, documentation, and reporting. They are known to "stretch"for either the fourteen days of acute rehab allowed and/or the hundred or more days for ongoing rehab care. Some play by the rules and some don't, and some do both depending on circumstances. With that information in mind, this is what many people in your situation might do.

"Let's take a typical husband in your position as an example. He takes his wife home from the care facility. After that he has to figure out a way to have her admitted to an acute-care hospital— sometimes an event may create the hospital admission, like breaking a bone or developing pneumonia. If providence doesn't give him a reason for an acute-care hospital admission, he can call an ambulance and claim that his wife fell and was unconscious and now is totally incoherent. The ambulance people will have no reason or excuse to avoid transporting her to an emergency room, and the ER will admit that patient because of such factors as 'defensive medicine' (the technical term for covering their asses to protect themselves from malpractice), the monetary incentive from Medicare and other types of insurance, pressures from family members, and pressures by the hospital authorities to fill beds.

"As I said," I continued, "once the patient is in an acute-care hospital for three or more days, that patient will become eligible for Medicare rehab. That's what many people in your shoes decide to do; they can find medical professionals who will readily coach them along the way. You can think about it. Meanwhile, you would do well to think about your own peace of mind and well-being. You can accept the current status and make daily visits, but also look into spending your new free time into doing some of the things you haven't been able to do for a very long time. You've earned that small reward, since you've carried out your marriage vows and have taken care of your wife the best you could."

We talked about other social and political issues. In my religious upbringing it's called a *mitzvah* (good deed) to help someone unload to another human being without being judgmental. It isn't as easy as it sounds. Listening and providing knowledge, compassion, and empathy takes learning and patience. It can be very rewarding for the listener. But this man never called me back.

There's a well-worn saying that knowing history should help to prevent the repetition of errors. Or, in other words, it's unrealistic to expect different outcomes if you keep doing the same thing over and over again. Take the evolution of medical-commercial complexes, starting with nursing-home care and morphing into four general levels of care directed primarily at our aging population. These can be categorized as

1. *independent living*, which can be either at home or in a controlled environment;
2. *assisted living*, which requires minimal oversight;
3. *assisted living with skilled nursing care*, which is sometimes called "memory care"; and
4. *total required care*, which involves skilled nursing services; required assistance in daily-living activities such as bathing, dressing, and eating; and locked doors, monitors, cameras, and other forms of protection to prevent injury and/or death.

To meet these various needs we've seen the creation of rehabilitation facilities, group-home living, and large and small medical companies that have built complexes to handle all or part of the levels of care that are required (as outlined above). Legislators have tried to provide safeguards and oversight to protect those in need, but this requires continuous attention and action—something that seems to wax and wane relative to competing priorities within global societal-media worlds.

Several truths emerged early on in this industry's evolution: all facilities preferred clients who could pay out of pocket or those with high-paying insurance plans. Medicare was high on the list of good payers, but Medicaid (the welfare category) was at the bottom of the list. This situation still prevails and may affect the ability to find a bed for a person in need. Similarly, no facility wants a disruptive client, and to be frank, some can't deal with that kind of patient. That is why most places will have a face-to-face interview with the client before accepting him or her.

A diagnosis of Alzheimer's originally equated to potential behavioral problems (which is not universally true), and those very selective facilities bluntly and legally stated that "we will not accept patients with an Alzheimer's diagnosis." The immediate response was semantic manipulation. For instance, physicians used diagnoses that omitted the Alzheimer's label and instead used terms such as *mild cognitive impairment of unknown origin* or *dementia unspecified*, and facilities called *memory-care* sprang up all over the place. That way a patient could be admitted without diagnostic bias and if too disruptive the facility could subsequently evict the patient using the federal words "for their own safety"; indicating they were not equipped to safely provide what the patient needed. Necessity is the mother of creativity, and the promise of monetary reward gives that necessity a kick start.

Chapter VII

DOING GOOD TAKES GRIT

Courage, focus, drive, and passion: these add up to the belief that you can do something. If you are a caregiver/advocate, taking charge is a must. The pressure is unrelenting, and the arenas are often arbitrary or fortuitous. Learn all you can and continuously reevaluate yourself and your significant other. Remember the motto: "Trust, but verify." Attack problems at the roots: How accurate is the medical diagnosis? What is the true prognosis? Are the medications worth trying (i.e., risks versus benefits)? Who do I talk to?

To start my discussion, I have taken the liberty of reprinting an opinion piece by a highly qualified physician, Marwan Sabbagh, MD, director of the Alzheimer's and Memory Disorders division of the Barrow Neurological Institute, in Phoenix. This piece appeared in the *Arizona Republic* on Friday, November 27, 2015. Dr. Sabbagh had been with Banner Research, which I mentioned. earlier. Banner is a research program that has been in existence for approximately twenty-five years, and is located near Sun City, Arizona. I will present more material on Banner very soon. Barrow's Neurological Institute is an adjunct to St. Joseph's Hospital in Phoenix.

"Defeating Alzheimer's Is a Fight That Needs All of Us"

Alzheimer's Disease and Awareness Month is in November. It is easy to remember as it always follows Breast Cancer Awareness Month in which many breast cancer organizations have done such a great job increasing awareness. Ironically, and unbeknownst to many, Alzheimer's disease is far more common and the public concern is justifiably growing.

The statistics are staggering. Alzheimer's disease is now the fourth leading cause of death in the United States and is the only one in the top 25 diseases that has been steadily growing. Presently, the condition affects 5.4 million Americans and 150,000 in Arizona alone.

It is the leading cause of long term care placement and accounts for up to 60 percent of long term care insurance claims. Approximately $160 billion is spent annually in the United States for Alzheimer's disease-related costs and expenses and the condition affects one in 10 over the age of 65.

More than 100,000 die from Alzheimer's disease each year, and it's estimated that 14 million Americans will have the disease by the year 2050—affecting one in eight Baby Boomers.

Interestingly, a national survey of 1,000 baby boomers finds that they are clearly not ready emotionally, physically, or financially to deal with Alzheimer's disease in their own future. The vast majority are extremely concerned about the potential impact of the disease on their health, quality of life, and finances as well as on the health care system.

More than 90 percent of survey respondents said they would either be unprepared or find life "not worth living" if diagnosed with the illness. Eighty percent of respondents said their savings would not be sufficient to cover the cost of care while 84 percent feel that more should be done to prioritize treatment and research to fight the debilitating disease.

Surrounding the illness is the sense of futility widely held by caregivers, patients and practitioners alike. There is a collective sense that nothing can be done once you're diagnosed with the condition. As a geriatric neurologist who has dedicated my life to taking care of people with Alzheimer's disease and other forms of dementia, I can say that medical science has advanced a lot more than most people are aware and that there is hope.

In point of fact, we can now diagnose Alzheimer's disease in individuals with 90 percent accuracy. There are groundbreaking treatments that are being developed, that if successful and approved, could be available as early as 2018. These treatments could offer real meaningful progress in slowing down the disease.

Adding to this sense of hope is the knowledge that physicians and scientists in Arizona are leading the national and global fight against Alzheimer's disease. Through Barrow Neurological Institute and the Arizona Alzheimer's Research Consortium, huge advances are being made including innovative ways to diagnose, detect and attack the disease as well as research studies that are targeting the changes in the brain before the onset of symptoms.

However, to see a future without Alzheimer's disease, the medical and research communities need engagement and participation from those who are affected by or at risk for the illness. Thus, waiting for others to participate delays advances for everyone.

It took unrelenting perseverance on my part to discover Banner Sun Health Research Institute, even though it's been around for over twenty-five years. Nevada has no such research program, although one medical center said it had hired two people and intended to develop such a program. This most likely won't happen in my lifetime. I will discuss my experience with Banner, which has been excellent, and I am including copies of the institute's informational fliers below. If you are a caregiver/advocate in Arizona, I highly recommend that you contact them. If you live in another state, start calling to see if you can locate a similar program. I can't stress enough the importance of this type of program to further our understanding of neurodegenerative diseases.

The Banner Research Institute is free of charge to Arizona residents of six or more consecutive months. My wife qualified, since she had been permanently entered into a skilled-nursing group home for six months following her fall that resulted in wrist and hip fractures. After the six months she was transferred to a skilled-nursing memory-care facility in Scottsdale.

We provided all of the family and personal medical histories to start the enrollment process for Banner Research. She and I both participated in extensive, periodic medical follow-ups that included evaluating any changes in movement abilities, cognition, mood, balance, medications, and relevant laboratory testing. The program is designed to give a clear picture of her clinical progression (good and bad) as well as possible entry into a research protocol (if appropriate). Finally, when she passes away, a postmortem will be conducted within a few hours of her death. Her chart at her memory-care facility has the directive clearly displayed and the number to call around the clock.

The postmortem pathological findings by a qualified neuropathologist (a pathologist who specializes in brain diseases) will be added to her clinical record for review and correlations. Some researchers refer to this process as "biodata banking." In order to validate our clinical diagnosis and understanding, we must have the postmortem findings. As of the writing of this book (in 2016), no working neuropathologist is available anywhere in the entire state of Nevada. Our clinical (living) diagnoses are not always correct. It is a vital learning process and, as Dr. Sabbagh's article states, "Waiting for others to participate delays advances for everyone." Researchers need people with positive family histories and those with an active disease. I hope the media focuses more attention than it has on making patients and families aware of the opportunities and the necessity of participating, as well as on getting doctors to participate and make referrals.

Dr. Sabbagh had not yet joined the Barrow Neurologic Institute when I called the institute; he was still at Banner at the time. The person I spoke to at Barrow told me: "We do not have such a program at this time. We can evaluate your wife for a diagnosis and possibly suggest treatment."

I told him that we already had all of that. I then called the Arizona branch of the Mayo Clinic, but they gave me the same answer. Neither mentioned Banner, which is strange, since some of both groups' neurologists do participate in patient evaluations for the Banner Research Program. I did leave a message for Dr. Sabbagh at his new office at Barrow about the need for better communication and participation among physicians and their groups.

I lucked out when I called the neurology department at Arizona State University. The head of the department mentioned Banner and gave me the group's phone number. It's free, funded, and staffed. It needs more aggressive media promotion, but this won't happen by itself.

For more information on Alzheimer's disease treatment and clinical trials, visit www.thebarrow.org.

And below is Banner's two-page flier.

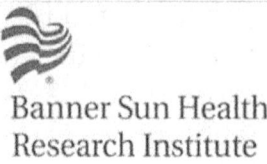

Banner Sun Health
Research Institute

Banner Sun Health Research Institute

Brain & Body Donation Program

Banner Sun Health Research Institute invites interested persons to partner with us in search of causes and cures for some of the most debilitating neurodegenerative diseases. Unfortunately, the underlying mechanisms of certain complex diseases are not well understood. The complexity of these diseases makes it important for scientists to have access to tissue in order to make scientific breakthroughs. Have you considered being a part of the Brain & Body Donation Program at Banner Sun Health Research Institute?

Why should I participate in the Brain and Body Donation Program?

Help is needed to find a cure for degenerative brain diseases that currently affect you and might affect your loved ones in the future. Participation in the Brain and Body Donation Program allows researchers to better understand the cause and progression of these diseases. Comparing diseased tissue and normal tissue will bring researchers much closer to finding crucial answers.

How do I enroll?

Participation requires filling out forms, providing consent to participate, listing current medications and a detailed medical/family history. We also ask for your permission to contact your primary care physician, and possibly other physicians, to obtain your medical records.

Once these forms are completed and returned to us, we will contact you to confirm your enrollment.

What will happen after I enroll?

As part of the program participants must undergo annual assessments which may include:

- Testing of learning, memory, concentration, language and neurological status

- A medical and family history update

- A movement function test

- A smell test

We understand that your time is valuable, and we will make every effort to schedule these appointments at your convenience. All information provided will help researchers target strategies for earlier diagnosis and to develop potential treatments.

In addition, your family will receive a free autopsy report within 9-12 months of the donation.

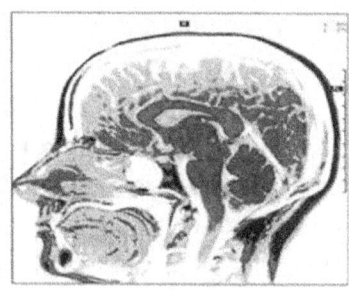

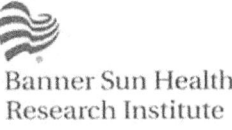

**Banner Sun Health
Research Institute**

Commonly Asked Questions

Will participation in this program cost the donor or their family members anything?

There is no cost to participants or their family for any part of the research or the autopsy report. If the participant chooses the whole body donation option, cremation is provided **at no cost** to the family.

What effect will brain donation have on funeral arrangements?

If brain donation only is chosen, it has no effect on funeral arrangements. It does not delay preparing the body for funeral, and the techniques used allow for an open-casket funeral. Whole body donation requires cremation and because of time restrictions to obtain brain tissue, may limit visitation for family and friends.

Can we still use our family funeral director?

Yes. After autopsy, the deceased can be sent to the funeral home of your choice.

What diseases or conditions are being researched through the tissue donation program?

Alzheimer's disease and Parkinson's disease.

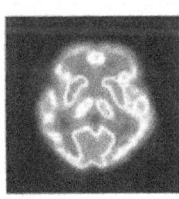

Do you collaborate with others?
The Brain and Body Donation Program at Banner Sun Health Research Institute collaborates with researchers and doctors from other institutions. These include members of the **Arizona Alzheimer's Consortium, Arizona Biomedical Research Commission, Michael J. Fox Foundation, NIH, Parkinson's Study Group and National Parkinson's Foundation.**

About Our Research Institute

Since its founding in 1986, scientists at non-profit Banner Sun Health Research Institute have earned an international reputation for breakthroughs in some of the most debilitating age-related diseases. The Institute's scientists have uncovered clues to those diseases through countless experiments utilizing tissue and data obtained through the brain and body donation program.

Scientists here are making history researching prevention and treatments in the fields of **Alzheimer's disease, Parkinson's disease and cardiovascular disease.**

Take a Tour

On the first Tuesday of every month, the public is invited to learn more about exciting progress in research during a 90-minute guided tour of the world-renowned Banner Sun Health Research Institute. Space is limited, call to register.

Contact us

For questions and information about the Brain and Body Donation Program call **623-832-6528 or 623-832-6511**

For more information about Banner Sun Health Research Institute, participation in one of our clinical trials, or to schedule a tour, please call **623-832-5328.**

www.BannerSHRI.com

10515 W. Santa Fe Drive, Sun City, Arizona, 85351

Before I comment on Dr. Sabbagh's article, let me repeat that my finding of Dr. Sabbagh and the Banner Sun Health Research Institute was the result of persistence and pure luck. As stated, Nevada has no such resource. The aforementioned Lou Ruvo Brain Center (part of the Cleveland Clinic), in southern Nevada, stated in its fall 2015 magazine (*New Thinking*, page 10) that "New

Cleveland Clinic biorespository will boost brain health research." That sounded great! But when I called the clinic, no one knew anything about the article or the status of that project. I get very upset when the media fails to check facts (and I'm being very kind here) and promotes false perceptions. I also become irate with the practice at the clinic of blocking any direct contact with its staff physicians. It is frustrating and incomprehensible, to say the least.

When I called Banner in Arizona, in contrast, I was readily connected to its director, Thomas G. Beach, MD, and we had a very professional and personal conversation. I bring this up because we cannot expect to attain the best research efforts or health-care delivery unless people set aside their egos and personal agendas for the greater good. I say God bless all of the physicians, allied-health professionals, and lay founders, supporters, and volunteers who have made the Arizona neurological programs a reality. This will require fine tuning, but these programs are models for excellent, effective, dedicated, and targeted research that every state should emulate.

Now let me comment on Dr. Sabbagh's article in the *Arizona Republic*. I am not criticizing Dr. Sabbagh's intentions or expertise; he is sincere, his advice is constructive, and his statistics are accurate. But he is speaking about his institution and about Arizonans. When he states that "medical science has advanced a lot more than most people are aware and that there is hope," I believe he is speaking more as a dedicated researcher in a very well-qualified neurological center. I still consider myself to be someone who shares the "sense of futility widely held by caregivers, patients and practitioners alike."

I say this knowing that we might make the patient more comfortable by playing music, surrounding him or her with "memory lane" photos and personal items, taking good care of the person's feeding and hygiene needs, and perhaps using mood-altering medications when appropriate. As I've mentioned elsewhere, however, I do not believe a credible case has been made for using Namenda or Aricept (or its patch equivalent, Exelon), and although promising ideas produce glimmers of hope, the definitive "big breakthrough" could be years away, as has been the case with other degenerative diseases.

Dr. Sabbagh also states that "In point of fact, we can now diagnose Alzheimer's disease in individuals with 90 percent accuracy." While that may well be true at his institutes, it is not true in the rest of our nation or elsewhere in the world. In that regard, researchers have shown many times that we are wrong at least 30 percent of the time if we look for specific imaging markers and autopsy findings. Many times the autopsy reveals the presence of the Lewy bodies we discussed earlier (which are not seen on any imaging we currently have) as the culprit; we also don't know much about them, so we refer to them simply as "abnormal proteins." Or the autopsy may simply reveal that microvascular strokes have occurred, which refers to the failure of small blood vessels in the brain. These strokes are similar to the circulatory problems that people often experience in the heart and/or with kidney circulation. This is why we need nationwide programs such as the Banner Research model, which not only tracks the necessary details during a patient's life but follows up with the patient after his or her death to acquire valuable postmortem information. People who enroll in the Banner program are indeed points of light at the end of the tunnel. Their dedication, integrity, and perseverance is admirable.

CHAPTER VIII

THE NAKED TRUTH

As our founding forefathers stated, some truths are self-evident, whether it be life, liberty, and the pursuit of happiness or the pursuit of a healthy lifestyle. Genetics defines the nuts and bolts, but how it all comes together to form a working human being can definitely be influenced by how we exercise, sleep, and play; how and what we eat and drink; and the ways in which humans in general pollute our air, water, and earth. Keep in mind, however, that there are those who would readily sell you things that have no proven value. Buyer beware.

Take the category of play: name a few popular sports like football, soccer, and skiing. We take some of our most genetically well-endowed people and have them compete against one another to the point of causing serious, crippling injuries and even death.

Sure, when the media gets involved, the respective sports industry tells us how much safer it has made its particular sport thanks
to the use of protective equipment and protocol adjustments. You
can draw your own conclusions. For me, high risks still prevail, and
introducing children to the benefits of exercise and sports must
include a serious understanding of the negatives involved.

The same goes for the food, nutrition, supplement, and additive
industries. You might see a media figure like Larry King interviewing
a woman with the title "doctor" but deliberately neglecting to say
what kind of doctor she is. She tells him how great her product is
for allegedly improving her patients' performances, while he leans
his chin against his hand and looks at her in rapt concentration. At
one time he was touting a product called Garlique, which was said
to convert your heart into a Cadillac-style engine. Why doesn't the
FDA have the authority to close such manufacturers down (with
stiff penalties, to boot)? In my opinion, they and others are knowingly selling pure crap. If you're really interested, ask your elected
representatives. You can corner these politicians for an answer.

I remember the saying, "Hope springs eternal." For some,
hope is a necessity. We need to embrace the concept of "We can
do better," but it has to be rooted in reality. Indeed, the greatest advancements have been achieved when we set aside egos,
greed, indifference, and personal and group differences. In health
care, for example, we desperately need tort reform and the ability
to buy health insurance across state lines. (Congress passed laws
to allow congress people that privilege, but the same congress
people deny it to the people who elected them.) We also need
an expansion of the FDA to meaningfully regulate food additives and supplements. (*Meaningfully* here refers to very clearly
defined rules and regulations—with significant penalties for rule
breakers—and no loopholes.)

One of my greatest disappointments is related to the lack of
honest oversight of the frustratingly impenetrable and self-serving
behemoth that is the US health-care industry. If families and

patients do not have honest, knowledgeable advocates they are in deep trouble, especially if that lack of advocacy is coupled with limited financial resources. Let's take a few examples.

1. Medicare provides limited coverage in skilled-nursing assisted-living care, and that care is tied to being hospitalized for acute care: that is, a direct transfer after at least three days in the acute-care hospital.
2. Similarly, those with long-term-care insurance need to read their policies very closely, since many policies have limitations that lessen the policy's value.
3. Everyone should become familiar with what Medicaid means; it is intended for those who are considered to be living in poverty.
4. Similarly, poverty-level veterans (and their families) of World War II and the Korean and Vietnam Wars should check into VA aid and attendance pension benefits.
5. Medicare is the federally funded health-care plan. It does have early (at any age) disability benefits if the person qualifies. It is best to hire a lawyer who specializes in those benefit evaluations, but make sure that you pay nothing unless the lawyer is successful; payment would then be taken as a preagreed fee.

Care in skilled-nursing assisted-living facilities runs at least $5,000 a month, plus extras for medications; acute-care problems such as infections, falls, etc.; and hygiene care such as foot care and basic grooming.

Dr. Lisa Rosenberg, MD, a geriatrician in southern Nevada, sums up the challenges of caring for aging patients:

Geriatricians serve as the primary care providers for these older patients. We treat common diseases affecting older adults, and help to balance the benefit and burden of treatments. We also help manage other issues, such as chronic pain, mobility and falls, memory loss, incontinence, *many of which can be related to medication side effects*. (Emphasis added.)

Rosenberg also evaluates older people's ability to care for themselves (such as preparing meals, bathing, and dressing); she also screens for driving fitness and addresses any other changes to patients' independence.

As Dr. Rosenberg pointed out in the quote above, many medical problems may be iatrogenic in nature (i.e., doctor caused) and may be the result of side effects from medication. To make matters even more frustrating, the medications that are prescribed (or self-selected) are too often totally inappropriate; namely, there is and was no credible evidence to justify their use and/or adequate attention was not given to possible negative drug interactions.

I've already voiced my opinion that Namenda and Aricept should both be removed from the list of approved drugs for any type of dementia. This is why an article titled "America the Medicated" in a publication called *The Real Truth* (October/November 2015) caught my attention. I advise you in advance that this is a religion-based publication and I do not agree with many of its alleged religious correlations on other subjects. But I do believe that this article is well written and factual and that it lends more credence to the notion of the responsible prescribing and ingestion of both prescribed and over-the-counter substances. I also favor very stiff penalties for those who ignore the responsibilities that should be associated with substance promotion and availability. To quote my daughter, you don't make a deal with the devil to balance a budget.

Below are a few quotes from "America the Medicated."

Turn on any television across America and you will lightly glimpse one of the 80 of these that air hourly on stations across the nation. Commercials featuring families on fishing trips or prancing through fields, co-workers golfing or discussing the latest news over hearty salads, couples dancing, walking dogs, enjoying romantic candlelight dinners, or side by side in bathtubs overlooking the sunset—even glowing butterflies flitting from person to person to help them sleep. At first glance, such clips seem to advertise the great outdoors or healthy eating. In reality, though, they showcase what has become a staple of American life: prescription medications.

Behind these happy images, warnings are softly rattled off. One commercial for a self-injection medication for clearer skin ends with an announcer listing side effects far more concerning than the condition itself: "Serious sometimes fatal infections and cancers, including lymphoma, have happened, as have blood, liver and nervous system problems, serious allergic reactions, and new or worsening heart failure…

Such warnings are often tied to drugs to treat depression, diabetes, arthritis, osteoporosis, erectile dysfunction disorder, high cholesterol, fibromyalgia, and the list goes on.

Despite dire warnings from the drug companies themselves, more than 70 percent of Americans—223 million—take at least one prescription drug. Over 50 percent, about 160 million, take two prescription pills regularly.

Direct-to-consumer drug commercials are only permitted in the United States and New Zealand. And pharmaceutical companies in the US take full advantage of this ability, with many spending more than $4 billion a year on ads.

At this point I should mention that Congress was at one point considering outlawing direct-to-consumer commercials, but the powerful pharmaceutical lobby staved off the threat by promising that it would self-regulate. Self-regulation never happened, and the interest died (no pun intended). Back to the article.

Then there are drugs for the more than one in five people in America who have been diagnosed with a host of behavioral or mental issues—bipolar disorder, schizophrenia, obsessive-compulsive disorder, depression, aggression, attention deficit disorder, and mood instability. Each year, Americans spend more than $18 billion on antipsychotics, $11 billion on anti-depressants, and $7 billion on drugs to treat ADHD [attention-deficit/hyperactivity disorder].

The American Psychological Association expressed concerns regarding these figures and the possible "use of powerful antipsychotic drugs by elderly nursing home residents and the prescription stimulants to children who have been misdiagnosed with ADHD."

Dependence on medication has led to unintended consequences. Prescription drugs resulted in 22,767 deaths and 1.4 million emergency room visits in 2013, according to the most recent available data from the CDC [Centers for Disease Control and Prevention].

To one degree or another, everyone involved is responsible for the rise in the reliance on prescription medications, starting with the companies themselves, moving on to legislators who show everything from no interest to conflict of interest, and finally to physicians, care facilities, and sham oversight committees. I've given you my experience related to my wife and other patients in Arizona and Nevada, respectively. I wrote detailed documentation on deliberate fraud, abuse, and malpractice and submitted it to Medicare, United Health (my secondary insurance), the physician, and the care-facility licensing boards in both states. I have over half a century of experience in health care. I know fraud, abuse, and malpractice when it happens. Medicare gives everything to subcontractors who have no skin in the game and consequently rubber stamp everything. There is absolutely no accountability with any of these entities, and I have an inch-thick file on my wife's case to prove it. I have another case that served as the basis for an unpublished book manuscript titled *You the Jury.* In that case, a woman came within a breath of losing her life due to blatant malpractice by a doctor of osteopathy in southern Nevada and the associated denial of hospital-acquired infection due to MRSA (methicillin-resistant *Staphylococcus aureus*), even though the diagnosis was documented by a leading infectious-disease expert in southern Nevada.

Nothing will change unless you, the public, take ownership. For example, next time candidates are standing for election, ask them what *specifically* they will do to correct some of the problems I have discussed above to encourage prevention, treatment, and accountability. I would bet that most won't even bring the subjects up, let alone having specifics to address the problems.

CHAPTER IX

ACUTE CARE, PALLIATIVE CARE, HOSPICE CARE

It's important to understand the ever-changing terminology used in medical care. *Acute care* is relatively constant in that it involves a sudden onset of illness that requires immediate diagnosis and treatment. *Palliative care* has taken on an entirely new meaning as patients seek and receive pain and disease management that together allow added years with an acceptable quality of life. Palliative care may be important to consider for patients with a wide variety of diseases such as cancer, chronic heart failure, dementia, chronic lung disease, Parkinson's disease, multiple sclerosis, stroke, and advanced liver or kidney disease. Palliative care does not carry the time limit of prognosis that applies to *hospice care*, in which the patient is generally given six months or fewer before death. Some people group palliative care and hospice care into an *end-of-life* category, and Medicare has even created a payer code to encourage physicians to take time and discuss the following list (paraphrased here) with patients, caregivers, and advocates.

- Coordinate care with all of a patient's health-care providers.
- Provide emotional support for patients and their families.
- Discuss treatment options for both their primary disease and pain and symptom management.
- Choose the most appropriate setting for treatment, which might be the patient's home or a hospital or inpatient facility.
- Address any nonmedical issues that might arise, including financial status and job-related problems, insurance questions, and legal issues.

As a family physician who worked for thirteen years in a rural setting (1960–1973), many of these functions were automatically included by myself and by my primary-care colleagues. But with extraordinary medical advances and skyrocketing patient loads and costs, it has become virtually impossible for solo practitioners to find the time. It takes a team effort, which entails planning, motivation, and reasonable remuneration for the health-care providers. It also takes education and inclusion for the caregivers, advocates, and patients.

Chapter X

ONE FROM THE HEART

In my youth I looked a lot like my grandfather on my mother's side. Once I passed sixty-five I looked more like my dad. I can't complain about my genetic pool and I certainly am appreciative of a loving, disciplined, and sensitivity-oriented upbringing. I do not minimize the importance of liberal amounts of divine intervention, plain luck, or whatever else you want to call it. So when I am asked the frequent question, "How is it going?" I can only shrug and say, "It could be worse."

With our daughter's encouragement and the help of Kay Leslie Segal of Scottsdale and her excellent editing, I started to write a few introspective thoughts in the form of blogs on my website, www.doctorlenk.com. The "LenK" part refers my first name and last initial. I then went on to writing this book.

"Dad," she said, "you should write a small chapter titled 'One from the Heart.' It will make the book much more personal and would also give you more credibility as a caregiver. I know you'll cry during the writing of it, but that's healthy."

Our daughter is wonderfully endowed with creativity, which makes it virtually impossible to not listen to her when she speaks. I'll start this chapter with two of my blogs. I'll probably never stop crying (metaphorically speaking) because of the thoughts that never leave me. My current compromise with reality is essentially to lead a double life. The awareness, acceptance, and support of my entire family (and friends who know) makes it more workable, but it's still *strange* for a man who's been married and faithful for fifty-nine years. I am in a great relationship with a widow who lost her husband to a ten-year fight with aggressive Parkinson's. We share our past experiences and take comfort from our legacies, and she encourages the continuance of my undying, loving commitments to Joan. It's as good as it can be, since there are no perfect alternatives.

Blogs from the Website
www.doctorlenk.com

"Caregiver Frustration: An Open Letter"
March 2, 2014

This letter (slightly edited here for book format, as is the blog post that follows) was sent to the benefactor who fostered the creation of the Cleveland Clinic's Lou Ruvo Center for Brain Health in Las Vegas. I, like many caregivers, want help and hope for those to whom we provide care. As you will see, my frustration mounted when I encountered yet another dead end. If you are a caregiver, I hope this will help to warn you that trying to find help is a twisted and frustrating process, but you are not alone. Stay positive and passionate and you could prevail over the system.

Dear Mr. Ruvo: February 25, 2014
I do not enjoy being the bearer of negative commentary, but if not me, who else? You should know that what is advertised in your quarterly publication of *Keep Memory Alive* is not what is provided at the Cleveland Clinic. I am also informing you, in all fairness, that this is an open letter, which means that I will offer it for general publication and/or a blog on my website (www.doctorlenk.com). Too many caregivers (civilian and military, young and old) are given false hope—sometimes deliberately and sometimes inadvertently—but always with the same cruel, hope-crushing consequences.

When I received the spring 2014 publication from your establishment, I thought that perhaps my letter to you on June 13, 2013, might have led to the notice on page 22 of your publication, which I've quoted below. I had written to you about the serious lack of support services in southern Nevada, especially in cognitive therapy. You forwarded my letter to Dr. Cummings, MD, director of the clinic in Las Vegas, who conferred with Dr. Bernick, MD, his head of neurology. Dr. Cummings's response was essentially that my assessment was correct, but the clinic did not have money or space to address the problem of cognitive-therapy services. It really comes down to priorities and willingness to make the effort. Dr. Cummings did say that the clinic might hire an occupational therapist "when space and financial circumstances allow."

The following is from page 22 from the spring edition of *Keep Memory Alive*: "Group Therapy: One Concept. Two Options."

Group exercise classes conducted by a Cleveland Clinic physical therapist focus on maintaining function in the lives of Cleveland Clinic Lou Ruvo Center for Brain Health patients. Patients can choose between two classes:

1. Parkinson's disease exercise class: tailored to the movement symptoms of Parkinson's disease.
2. Group exercise class: a seated exercise class open to individuals with any neurodegenerative disorder.

I called the number that was provided in the publication (702-483-6000), but the person at the front desk did not know what I was talking about. I told the receptionist that I was a physician and that my wife had been seen by Dr. Bernick. The receptionist took the information and pulled up my wife's record. I referred her to page 22 of the publication. After several holds, the frustrated receptionist apologized and said that she would get back to me. (This was February 5, 2014.) Two days later I called and asked when they were planning to get back to me. She again apologized, and finally someone did call later that day and told me that I could only attend the 11:15 a.m. class, since the 12:30 p.m. class was for Parkinson's patients.

She suggested that I should simply bring my wife down and try the class out before paying the eighty dollars for a month's participation.

I arrived at 10:30 a.m. on February 25th (earlier than the suggested 10:45). No one knew what I was talking about. I showed them page 22. They asked us to wait in the lounge across from the reception desk. By 11:00 a.m., I inquired with the receptionist about the extensive wait.

"Oh," she replied. "There must be people out there by now. It's the building right behind you. In fact, you can follow the man who just went in to use the restroom; he's in the group."

The man who had just gone into the restroom was obviously a Parkinson's patient, which meant that he should have been in the 12:30 group, according to what I had originally been told. I took my wife to the building that the receptionist had pointed out. The facility was set up for some sort of social function, which included an open bar. The people in charge were very pleasant and directed me to a gathering of chairs in the courtyard. The therapist showed up at exactly 11:17 a.m. I went up and introduced myself and explained that my wife was there to try the group exercises. She looked at me as if I were speaking a foreign language. I made it very clear that my wife did not have muscle weakness, balance problems, etc.

Her reply: "Have her try it anyway. She might like it, or you can come back at 12:30."

My next questions for the clinic were: What were the credentials of the therapist? Was she really a trained therapist, or was she just another fitness trainer? Did any of the professors oversee the program at regular intervals? Was this another example of public-relations window dressing?

I drove my wife home and made her lunch: another day in the life of a caregiver.

"Hotel Paradise"
April 2, 2015

On Tuesday, March 31, 2015, the *Wall Street Journal* wrote that "According to the Alzheimer's Association, about 40% of caregivers for dementia (patients with cognitive problems) suffer from depression. Caring for a dementia patient is typically 'the most negatively impactful and the most challenging type of caregiving,' said Richard Schulz, psychiatry professor at the University of Pittsburg. 'The symptoms are constantly in front of you. That takes a big toll.'"

An estimated fifteen million relatives and friends help with an estimated 5.3 million Alzheimer's-type patients, not to mention the millions who take care of all of the other types of dementias, such as those associated with Parkinson's disease, Lewy bodies, or circulatory problems. Again from the *WSJ* article: "Primary caregivers change diapers and feed and bath their husbands and wives, mothers and fathers. They juggle jobs and other family responsibilities, and deal with often exorbitant expenses and difficult end-of-life decisions." So, you might ask: Why the title for this blog in my caregiver series?

After ten years as my wife's primary home caregiver, primary-care physician, and the holder of the power of attorney, she lost her balance in November 2014 and fell while visiting family in Arizona. She fractured her right wrist and right hip. We navigated the acute medical care as well as the rehabilitation process and arrived at the point of deciding where and what skilled-nursing facility we would try. "Trying" is a key concept for all of us. Nothing should be cast in concrete. I constantly remind myself to consider and adapt: I should seek and accept help.

A suburb of Scottsdale called Paradise Valley has a ten-person group home. The area is considered to be upscale, akin to Beverly Hills, California, on the West Coast or Scarsdale, New York, on the East Coast. The group facility is impeccably maintained, superbly supervised, and it has the most caring, compassionate staff imaginable. My wife's primary needs have been met, and then some: daily medications; daily hygiene, food, and fluids; and a very upbeat and tranquil ambiance. This is something that is not taught but is shared by the entire carefully selected staff. This is why we metaphorically named the desert oasis "Hotel Paradise" for its location and services.

Being firm yet patient and prioritizing the needs of our loved ones is especially tough when making caregiving decisions. Hotel Paradise hosts ten totally different personalities, each of whom have varying diagnoses and medical needs. For example, some residents have call buttons on their person. My wife can't handle one. She either misplaces it or pushes the button randomly when she doesn't really need help. The staff uses strategically placed monitors and also tells her to call loudly if she needs help. She is constantly reminded to use her walker. I have repeatedly reassured the staff that I know she may fall sometime in the future, even with people standing around her. As I've noted earlier in this book, this actually did happen, in November 2014, when she fell and suffered her fractures. I, and several others, were right next to her and could not catch her in time.

This raises the concept of flexibility in our thinking and reacting. To paraphrase creed of Alcoholics Anonymous: Give us the wisdom to recognize that which we cannot control and the power and means to manage the changes we can control. Take comfort in knowing that we will never be 100 percent in control. While it's very difficult to control our emotions and accept our imperfections at controlling our loved ones' (and our own) mortality, doing so can certainly translate into better care for the caregivers and their recipients.

It was April Fool's Day, 2015, and I joined my wife, who was finishing her late breakfast in the dining room of Hotel Paradise. It was indeed another spring day in paradise as we moved to the covered patio to voice whatever came to mind; snooze as gentle, citrus-blossom-scented breezes brushed our cheeks and fore-heads; or viewed the majestic contours of Mummy Mountain in the distance. We repeatedly marveled at the prolific desert foliage of red and white oleander, lush green citrus trees, and multicol-ored ground cover of lantana, bush morning glories, and other assorted mystery plants. Three other ladies were escorted out to join us. Who knows what, if anything, they were thinking as air-planes repeatedly crossed high in the Caribbean-blue sky. It was soothingly quiet, save for the faint trickle from a central fountain that was surrounded by more flowers. A desert dove balanced itself on the fountain's edge, took a sip, and nodded approval in our direction. The faces of my wife and her three companions were content and more mystical than the portrait of the smiling Madonna. Hotel Paradise was appropriately branded.

"More Thoughts from the Heart"

Understanding, flexibility, and initiative are essential for get-ting the most out of what life has to offer. This sounds simple, but it's far from it. A myriad of environmental factors take turns try-ing to influence the outcomes of the various traits and predispo-sitions that we inherit. Fatalists might say that it's all a roll of the dice: What will be will be. Others make educated decisions and then hope for the best, while far too many are distracted to even given it a thought.

Some compare life to making wine in that aging should make it better. It helps to know what makes the most of the aging pro-cess (and how we can make the most of it), and a little luck never hurts. After eight decades I have indeed accepted the notion that I have been a *loner*. It hasn't been a bad thing in terms of setting and achieving goals, but it did exact a price. I had to postpone, deny, or substitute social pleasures that many of my adolescent and young-adult peers were experiencing. Achieving goals pro-duced accolades from parents, friends, and mentors, however, and it did soothe the psyche and divert those fleeting moments of loneliness to the deeper recesses of my consciousness. As they say, "there is nothing that succeeds like success," and success can become addictive.

But what happens when those goal-seeking pressures and accomplishments cease to be necessary? Has the person developed other interests to occupy freed-up time and deliver enjoyment? Has he produced and nurtured a loving, productive family? Has she been able to create a sustainable economic retirement portfolio? Or, as is too often the case, will this person just go on to die a lonely death in the saddle, riding aimlessly across a barren, monotonous landscape? When the drive wanes and the need to achieve falls to the bottom of the priority list, memories may try to fill the idle moments. For the loner the deafening silence can be an awful challenge, especially at night when one is in bed alone.

Is it any wonder that the caregiver husband (in my case) may desperately crave companionship when his wife enters a nursing home or care facility and the caregiver, whether consciously or unconsciously, knows it is not going to get better? The marriage vows are being fulfilled, the wife is being cared for in the best way possible, but nagging questions battle the forces of guilt, reality, and denial.

Here is a narrative from a *Dear Abby* (written by Jeanne Phillips) column that relates to this topic.

Dear Abby:

My wife is in a nursing home and will be for a long time. While I was caring for her at home, I was very lonely. She wasn't there for me except to demand that I do this and that.

I did what I could to keep her happy, but nothing worked. I had no life of my own. My life was wrapped around her and doing the best to take care of her. I did all the chores that were required to keep the home running. Would it be wrong to find a woman friend to do a few things with, like have dinner or go

to a movie or just for a ride in the country or to the beach? My son thinks I shouldn't do this, but he doesn't know how lonely I am, nor do the other kids in the family.
—No Life of My Own

Dear No Life:

You're asking me a question no one can decide for you. Much depends on the quality of your marriage before your wife became ill. You promised to love and cherish her until death do you part. If she's still in her right mind you owe it to be there for her to the extent that you can—just as she would be if you were sick and in a nursing home.

You should discuss all of this with your children. Although it is important that you spend enough time with your wife to ensure that she's being well cared for, you are also entitled to have a life. Some husbands want to spend every possible minute at their wife's bedside, while others do what you are contemplating. Only you can look into your heart and decide what would be best for all concerned, because it may affect your entire family.

This certainly hit home for me, as it must have resonated with thousands of other caregivers in similar situations across our nation. I made my decision after ten years of caregiving at home and an additional year ensuring the best care possible in a group home and (eventually) in a memory-care facility. It's frustratingly painful for me to watch her gradually slipping into another world with only flickering memories to keep her company. She's getting the best medical and custodial care possible, and the children and grandchildren visit whenever possible. They appear to fully understand, as does their nanna. She smiles often, sleeps a lot, and accepts the help that is provided to her; she expresses no complaints.

I've discussed it with family as opportunities arise and, although each has most likely reached his or her own conclusions (along with possibly lingering unanswerable questions), the consensus seems to be one of acceptance that I have done a good job in fulfilling my marriage vows and that the final decisions are mine to make.

Interestingly, our youngest son, an anesthesiologist in Overland Park, Kansas, asked me if I wanted to meet a widow when I came to visit him and his family for the Jewish high holiday of Rosh Hashanah. I think he is particularly sensitive to the challenges of going it alone following an amiable divorce after thirteen years of marriage and three children who were still living at home. I told him I was interested, and we met for lunch and again in synagogue. One might infer from a religious-spiritual sense that the circumstance of the meeting was indeed sanctioned by religious blessings. Others might say that it was self-serving rationalization.

The attractive, accomplished woman in question is close to my wife's age, and I am the exact age of her husband, who had passed away three years earlier from the progressive ten-year toll of Parkinson's disease. He came from Brooklyn, and I was born in Brooklyn but grew up in nearby White Plains. She has four accomplished children who are the same age as my three children, and we both have numerous enjoyable grandchildren. We've spent many hours sharing wonderfully comparable memories and thoughts, and we have agreed to continue doing so as we go forward with new experiences to add even more memories. As is often said, caring is sharing. I've found it easy and wonderful to talk of things I've never shared with anyone; indeed, I've started to shed my loner mantle. She has expressed the same feeling. She says that I talk too much, and I promised to control this new-found freedom so that she can contribute her part to the union. We agree that nothing should be left unsaid between those who care enough to make life as rewarding and enjoyable as possible for ourselves, our families, and our friends. I will still be with my wife as she is today and will always have the wonderful memories of how she was. I will visit as often as necessary to ensure her care and will reaffirm my love and presence to her despite her flickering comprehension. As a movie title once proclaimed, this is *As Good As It Gets*—with an added new beginning.

EPILOGUE

A farmer knows that clearing the land for cultivation requires ongoing weeding, fertilizing, and oversight. Engineers stress ongoing maintenance and repair for the longevity and maximum performance of their creations. Ensuring a safe and healthy workplace is no different. All attempts to improve our lives depend on continuously ensuring integrity, commitment, and performance.

We are not born biologically equal, nor are we exposed to uniform challenges. People have attempted to create general guidelines for daily living: Ten Commandments–type principles to live by. Too often, however, the human character and happenstance dictate less-than-worthy or desired outcomes.

I have been blessed with a life of incredible privilege and accomplishment. I was able to sort out, with bumps along the way, various questions of heritage, self-image, and purpose. I replaced shyness and naïveté with confidence and understanding. On balance I know that I've made my parents proud, I did more good than harm, and our children and grandchildren have taken our examples and teachings to higher levels.

I wrote this book to show that everyone can contribute to the betterment of society, even if this is difficult to do at times. We can't all amass fortunes, leave endowments, or create monuments, but we can strive for integrity, empathy, compassion, and forgiveness: things that give hope and meaning to our brief journey on Earth.

References and Further Reading

Neurology Now is a free publication for individuals with neurologic conditions, their caregivers, and their families: excellent materials for nonprofessionals and professionals alike that can be helpful in directing caregivers to other resources.

NeurologyNow.com
1-800-422-2681
333 Seventh Avenue, 19th floor
New York, NY 10001

For a full listing of patient organizations, go to bit.ly/NN-patientoreganizations.com. I highly recommend that you look at the April/May 2016 issue, which has two great articles, on suicide and troubleshooting sleep problems. These are tremendously important for caregivers and patients alike.

Below is a partial list of references from *Neurology Now* that covers a multitude of conditions.

Parkinson's Disease and Movement Disorders
American Parkinson Disease Association
apdaparkinson.org
800-223-2732

Foundation for PSP, CBD, and Related Brain Diseases
curepsp.org
800-457-4777

International Essential Tremor Foundation
essentialtremor.org
888-387-3667

The Michael J. Fox Foundation for Parkinson's Research
michaeljfox.org
800-708-7644

Lewy Body Dementia Association
lbda.org
404-935-6444

National Parkinson Foundation
parkinson.org
800-473-4636

Parkinson's Disease Foundation
pdf.org
800-457-6676

The Parkinson's Institute and Clinical Center
thepi.org
800-655-2273

Tremor Action Network
tremoraction.org
510-681-6565

Post-Polio Syndrome
Post-Polio Health International
post-polio.org
314-534-0475

Rare Diseases
Adult Polyglucosan Body Disease Research Foundation
apbdrf.org
646-580-5610

Global Genes Project
globalgenes.org
949-248-7273

The National Institutes of Health (NIH) Genetic and Rare Diseases
Information Center
rarediseases.info.nih.gov
301-251-4925; 888-205-2311

National Organization for Rare Disorders
rarediseases.org
203-744-0100; 800-999-NORD (6673)

Stroke
American Stroke Association: A Division of the American Heart
Association
strokeassociation.org
888-4STROKE (478-7653)

National Stroke Association
stroke.org
800-STROKES (787-6537)

Traumatic Brain Injury
Brain Injury Association of America
biausa.org
800-444-6443

Trigeminal Neuralgia (TN)
The Facial Pain Association
fpa-support.org
800-923-3608

Living with TN
livingwithtn.org
(No telephone number listed.)

As you can see, many references deal with the same disease process, and vast resources may be found for many other diseases. While caregivers/advocates can get answers to questions that are specific to their needs, it does take a lot of perseverance; in some cases, the answers and options may fall short of expectations. The following list discusses other references that should help caregivers/advocates in their quest.

VA aid and attendance pension benefit. This VA pension benefit is available to veterans and surviving spouses who require regular care and assistance based on certain health conditions. This is a tax-free benefit that is paid directly to the claimant to help offset the cost of care expenses that are provided either in the veteran's home, an assisted-living community, independent living (in limited situations), or in a nursing home. Contact your local VA center and remember that as with any governmental agency, services may vary from area to area and at various times. If you do not find answers and/or appropriate help, it is your duty to report the problem to your elected officials and the media. They are obligated to carry out legal mandates; all of us have to be proactive to see that they do just that.

Banner Sun Health Research Institute. This is a nonprofit brain and body donation program that is available to residents of Arizona. There is no out-of-pocket expense to participants. It is a vital program for patients, caregivers, and researchers who are dedicated to understanding the causes and cures for some of the most debilitating of neurodegenerative diseases. Other states may have comparable programs. I strongly urge investigating, understanding, and participating in similar programs for those who live outside Arizona. Address: 10515 W. Santa Fe Drive, Sun City, AZ 85351. 623-832-6511.

Hospice services. An excellent article that put to rest a host of nonexistent beliefs relative to hospice care was published in the *Prime View*, a division of the *Las Vegas Review Journal*, on Wednesday, June 5, 2013. A must read that is partially paraphrased below.

For good reason, Las Vegas is proud of the Nathan Adelson Hospice. It was the first hospice west of the Mississippi and the second in the United States. The founder, Nathan Adelson, was a grocer and father of Merv Adelson, a TV mogul and philanthropist. Merv Adelson and Irwin Molaski were business partners in various Las Vegas construction projects, notably Sunrise Hospital. Although Nate Adelson had no hospital administrative experience, his son Merv put him in that position at the hospital, where he proved to be very effective and extremely well liked. He later developed pancreatic cancer and had a very difficult time before passing away. Merv thought that there had to be a better way of making end-of-life challenges better for both patient and families. Adelson and partner Irwin Molaski eventually built the Nathan Adelson Hospice on donated land. The original concept accepted patients for in-house end-of-life care whom doctors had certified as having approximately six months to live. That is no longer strictly adhered to, and the center has also developed the capacity to offer home-care visits. No one is turned away for lack of insurance or finances. The center will accept Medicare and other forms of insurance and it pools that funding with extensive philanthropic support. The center is truly nonprofit, extremely ethical, and is very well run. I know of no one who meets the center's medical criteria ever being turned away.

I emphasize this last point, because over the years many care providers in southern Nevada (at one time I was told up to ninety) have promoted themselves as being hospice care or other titles or subtitles such as memory care, skilled-nursing care, rehabilitative care, or chronic care. The fact is that they are strictly for-profit enterprises and have considerably varying degrees of professional expertise. In southern Nevada, I strongly suggest consulting with Nathan Adelson Hospice before looking elsewhere. This is also true for every part of the United States. For example, the woman I knew in Overland Park, Kansas, whose husband had progressive Parkinson's disease was adamant to the end that he should remain at home. She honored his wish, brought in help, and modified the interior of their house as needed. In the last two to three years her hospice did do periodic home visits and did accept whatever insurance was available. Caregivers and advocates have to continuously look at options for themselves and their persons in need. That includes the next category, Medicare and Medicaid.

Medicare and Medicaid. Medicare is the well-intentioned federally mandated medical retirement safety net. Medicaid is the program that is primarily intended for the poor; it is state funded, with additional federal funding. States differ in how they run their Medicaid programs. If a person is on Medicaid and needs hospital care, doctor care, or skilled-nursing facilities, as well as medications, Medicaid will cover what the patient needs, *but* problems do arise when a Medicaid patient tries to find goods and services that will accept what Medicaid pays. Some physicians will flat-out refuse to accept Medicaid patients and/or Medicare patients.

Caregiver facilities will usually accept Medicaid clients but they may play games with bed availability when they have insured clients who are waiting to get in. Medicare subcontracts just about everything, including compliance and oversight. I've had personal experience in filing airtight complaints of fraud and abuse— remember, I have had over fifty years of professional experience and I definitely know fraud and abuse when it occurs—and over 95 percent of the time, those valid complaints are summarily dismissed. This is why United Health Insurance reported an estimated $282 billion in fraud and abuse for Medicare in 2015, and the aforementioned former doctor/senator Tom Coburn of Oklahoma reported another $115 billion in fraudulent Medicare disability claims in 2015.

Examples of pure fraud can be seen any day on television in motorized wheel chairs, braces for every joint in the body, catheters and medications for diabetes, and other services such as oxygen supplies. I personally received a call from a medical-supply company in southern Nevada in which the caller asked if I would fill out prescriptions (without ever seeing the patient) for oxygen, medications, and braces. I also receive promotional gimmicks in the mail. Private entrepreneurs send mailers that look like genuine government informational items. They are not genuine. They are trying to get you into their data bank, along with your personal information. Call Medicare before you provide any information. One mailer came with my wife's name on it and the following heading: "Medicare Special Needs Plans: Do You Qualify?"

Right off the bat I asked myself how they got my wife's name and mailing address. They went on to say the following: "Dear Joan, as a Medicare Beneficiary in Clark County, NV, you may be eligible to receive benefits through a Medicare Special Needs Plan!"

Such scams go on to tell the recipient that he or she might be eligible for certain benefits; this one said, "To find out if you're eligible for a Medicare Special Needs Plan, simply complete the postage-paid card below. There is absolutely no cost or obligation for this information." If you then read the fine print, however, it tells you to verify the address on the reply card; they also explain that they are a licensed and certified representative of a Medicare group with a contract, and they add a few disclaimers. They are obviously a vested interest that is looking to make money from your taxes. This amounts to white-collar crime, in that they can (and do) play games with vetting your eligibility. This practice is condoned by our elected officials. We all need to treat public/government money as if it were our own, because it is.

Medicare does provide rehabilitative services following hospitalization for an acute medical or surgical problem. While the original intent is both commendable and straightforward, it did not take long for entrepreneurs to "game" the system. As a result, Medicare has tried to modify the mandates in order to minimize fraud and abuse. It's an ever-present game.

The caregiver/advocate must closely monitor what is being done relative to the options that Medicare provides. You have to continually be on top of things, or you will get short changed. Once the patient is discharged from the Medicare rehab services, he or she cannot be reinstated unless the patient reenters an acute-care hospital for three or more days; the process then starts anew. Medicare laws are very explicit about discharging and/or readmitting patients. It's the physician's responsibility to see that the rules are followed religiously.

Other Resources

I've listed several more resources below; using online search engines will save you a lot of driving around.

- Area Agency on Aging
- Family Caregiver Alliance (https://www.caregiver.org)
- National Alliance for Caregiving (http://www.caregiving.org)
- Caregiver Action Network (http://caregiveraction.org

Paul Singer is a political journalist for the Washington, DC, office of *USA Today*. His article in *USA Today* from Friday, June 12, 2015, page 2A, entitled "I'm Just a Guy Trying to Take Care of Mom," appears below. He uses a single reference, eldercare.gov, and sets up a treasure chest of leads, assuming that the caregiver/advocate has access to the Internet plus the skills and patience to find something close to what is required. Otherwise, the person has to find someone who can do it for him or her. I assume from his article that money was readily available once he found acceptable facilities and personnel. Without money, the outcome can be far more difficult than is described here. Here is Singer's narrative.

For Mother's Day this year I gave my mother an in-home care service.

Kind of a strange gift, but it is exactly what she wanted because it let her leave the nursing home where she was recuperating from a fall.

This is the fifth time my wife and I have been down this road with parents/elders, and it is always a shocking reminder of how complex our health care system is and how expensive elder care can be. [See *USA Today*, Wednesday, June 10, 2015: "How 15% of Seniors Account for Nearly Half of Medicare Spending."] We also discover each time that we are simply not prepared for it. Every day begins with a new mysterious challenge that we have never before considered.

The biggest problem we face in caring for our elders is that frequently they have no diagnosis other than *getting old*. And our medical system isn't built to handle that.

Each time we have embarked on elder care, we have discovered again how random the whole process is. We find the right caregiver largely by luck and by accident. This time it appears I have found a program that will provide what my other needs with government support that will make it affordable. [Side note: I'm sure Singer is referring to Medicare coverage for rehabilitation when transferred from a general hospital for medical or surgical/orthopedic care, assuming that protocols have followed.] But we must have spoken to two dozen providers and other experts before anybody mentioned this program to us. Turns out there is a website—eldercare.gov—that lists available resources around the country. Wish I had known that six months ago.

[Side note: I can't understand why health-care professionals such as physicians and social-service providers don't ensure that to be top priority for every case. Every patient or his or her advocate/caregiver should be required to sign a statement that these facts were explained completely and that the required paperwork was set in motion. Failure to do so should entail significant penalties and, of course, oversight has to be guaranteed.]

But this time I discovered again the remarkable acts of kindness bestowed on me by total strangers who know only this about me: I'm just a guy trying to take care of his mother.

For that fact alone, a government employee was willing to whisper in my ear a workaround for a bureaucratic hurdle her own agency had created, for that fact alone, a nurse slipped me a piece of paper with her phone number on it and said, "if anything goes wrong when you get her home, you call me." For that fact alone, the mechanic I had never met in a city where I don't live rearranged his schedule to fix my car so I could get back to my mother.

Perhaps this is the real path to a kinder, gentler nation. Approach everybody you encounter as somebody who is just trying to take care of his or her mother.

Odds are pretty good that it is true, or will be eventually. Among my peers, parent care is a primary topic of conversation these days. Once upon a time, we talked mostly about our jobs. Then we talked about weddings. Then we talked about real estate. Then we talked about children. Now we talk about parent care.

As a political reporter, I'm surprised parent care is not a bigger portion of our political conversation. Parent care is where a vast majority of our national health care costs go, and it is a heavy emotional and economic burden on nearly every family at some point. It also happens to be most directly relevant to people over the age of 40, who are the most reliable voters.

There is a raging argument over health care in this country, but it is generally a conversation about medical coverage for working-age people. We talk about the future of Social Security and Medicare, but those are addressed as fiscal issues and deficit drivers. The real issue is the practical, not the political. How are you taking care of your mother and how are you paying for it?

This is a question worth asking anybody running for office. I think it tells you something about them as a person. If they have never given a thought to parent care, they are either poor planners or callous children, or just not like the rest of us. If they are dealing with parent care, the question can be humanizing. I mean, I can disagree with your politics and your tactics and your interpretation of the Constitution, but once I discover you are just another guy trying to take care of his mother, I can have a little empathy for you. And I can offer the name of this really helpful service we found. And then we have some common ground to work from.

Another resource to read is *On My Own*, by Diane Rehm, in which the public radio host details her husband's battle with Parkinson's disease and her decision to support, as she puts it, the "right to choose to die," after her lawyer husband John Rehm was denied access to assisted suicide and starved himself to death. Rehm is candid about uninvited challenges in her married life, the very difficult decision to enter John into a care facility, and his silent-treatment response, her addiction to being wanted, and the waves of grief that still persisted after his passing.

Knowing about another's struggles, successes, and failures can give us direction and purpose.

ABOUT THE AUTHOR

Leonard Kreisler, MD, is from White Plains, New York. As well as being a board-certified consultant and speaker, he has taken on numerous other roles in his life.

- Cancer and genetic research, Roscoe B. Jackson Memorial Laboratory, Bar Harbor, Maine
- Bachelor of science degree, Allegheny College, Meadville, Pennsylvania
- Medical degree, University of Vermont School of Medicine
- Rotating internship, Grasslands Hospital, Westchester County, Valhalla, New York
- Captain, US Army Medical Corps, Fort Detrick and Fort Ritchie, Maryland
- Thirteen years' home/office solo general practice, Peekskill, New York
- Eighteen years as medical director of the Nevada Operations Office of the Department of Energy
- Chief of staff at the University Medical Center, Southern Nevada's teaching hospital
- Four years as a cruise-ship physician and speaker
- Special training in medical aspects of weapons of mass destruction (nuclear and biological)
- Board certifications in occupational medicine and family practice
- Former Federal Aviation Administration (FAA) medical examiner
- Certified Medical Review Officer (MRO) for drug surveillance and rehabilitation programs

Dr. Kreisler often thinks to himself, "what a wonderful world." He is what he calls a "seenager"—a senior teenager. He has everything that he wanted as a teenager, only sixty years later.

He doesn't have to go to school or work. He gets an allowance every month.

He has his own pad. He doesn't have a curfew. He has a driver's license and his own car. He has an ID that gets him into bars and the local whisky store. The people he hangs around with are not scared of getting pregnant. And he doesn't have acne.

Life is great. He has more friends that he should send this book to, but right now he can't remember their names.

To paraphrase Mark Twain (1835–1910), when age becomes an issue of mind over matter, if you don't mind, it doesn't matter.

NOTE: "What a wonderful world" and the photo of the couple in process of taking a dip was modified from an anonymous e-mail. I would have gladly given full credit and asked for permission to use the material but the owner could not be located. At the end of the day, a little humor is just what the doctor ordered. Thank you, whoever you are.

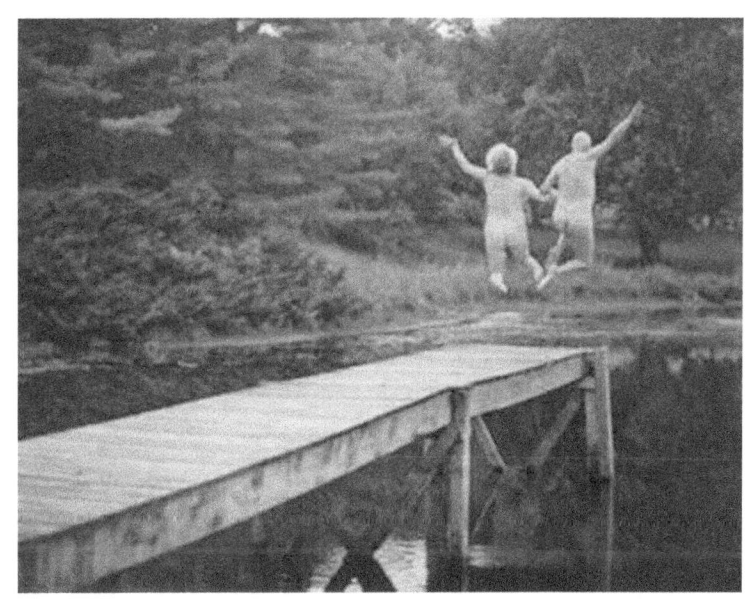

Photographer unknown

The end

www.ingramcontent.com/pod-product-compliance
Lightning Source LLC
Chambersburg PA
CBHW070321190526
45169CB00005B/1697